Reproductive Endocrinology

Editor

MICHELLE L. MATTHEWS

OBSTETRICS AND GYNECOLOGY CLINICS OF NORTH AMERICA

www.obgyn.theclinics.com

Consulting Editor
WILLIAM F. RAYBURN

March 2015 • Volume 42 • Number 1

ELSEVIER

1600 John F. Kennedy Boulevard • Suite 1800 • Philadelphia, Pennsylvania, 19103-2899

http://www.theclinics.com

OBSTETRICS AND GYNECOLOGY CLINICS OF NORTH AMERICA Volume 42, Number 1
March 2015 ISSN 0889-8545, ISBN-13: 978-0-323-35661-9

Editor: Kerry Holland
Developmental Editor: Stephanie Carter

Obstetrics and Gynecology Clinics (ISSN 0889-8545) is published quarterly by Elsevier Inc., 360 Park Avenue South, New York, NY 10010-1710. Months of issue are March, June, September, and December. Periodicals postage paid at New York, NY, and additional mailing offices. Subscription price per year is $310.00 (US individuals), $545.00 (US institutions), $155.00 (US students), $370.00 (Canadian individuals), $688.00 (Canadian institutions), $225.00 (Canadian students), $450.00 (foreign individuals), $688.00 (foreign institutions), and $225.00 (foreign students). To receive student/resident rate, orders must be accompanied by name of affiliated institution, date of term, and the signature of program/residency coordinator on institution letterhead. Orders will be billed at individual rate until proof of status is received. Foreign air speed delivery is included in all *Clinics* subscription prices. All prices are subject to change without notice. POSTMASTER: Send address changes to *Obstetrics and Gynecology Clinics*, Elsevier Health Sciences Division, Subscription Customer Service, 3251 Riverport Lane, Maryland Heights, MO 63043. **Customer Service: Telephone: 1-800-654-2452 (U.S. and Canada); 314-447-8871 (outside U.S. and Canada). Fax: 314-447-8029. E-mail: journalscustomerservice-usa@elsevier.com (for print support); journalsonlinesupport-usa@elsevier.com (for online support).**

Reprints. For copies of 100 or more of articles in this publication, please contact the Commercial Reprints Department, Elsevier Inc., 360 Park Avenue South, New York, New York 10010-1710. Tel.: 212-633-3874; Fax: 212-633-3820; E-mail: reprints@elsevier.com.

Obstetrics and Gynecology Clinics of North America is also published in Spanish by McGraw-Hill Interamericana Editores S.A., P.O. Box 5-237, 06500, Mexico; in Portuguese by Reichmann and Affonso Editores, Rio de Janeiro, Brazil; and in Greek by Paschalidis Medical Publications, Athens, Greece.

Obstetrics and Gynecology Clinics of North America is covered in MEDLINE/PubMed (Index Medicus), Excerpta Medica, Current Concepts/Clinical Medicine, Science Citation Index, BIOSIS, CINAHL, and ISI/BIOMED.

Contributors

CONSULTING EDITOR

WILLIAM F. RAYBURN, MD, MBA
Associate Dean, Continuing Medical Education and Professional Development, Distinguished Professor and Emeritus Chair, Obstetrics and Gynecology, University of New Mexico School of Medicine, Albuquerque, New Mexico

EDITOR

MICHELLE L. MATTHEWS, MD
Professor, Obstetrics and Gynecology; Director, 4th Year Medical Student Education; Associate Director, Reproductive Endocrinology, Carolinas HealthCare System, Charlotte, North Carolina

AUTHORS

ALICIA Y. ARMSTRONG, MD, MHSCR
Contraception Discovery and Development Branch, Eunice Kennedy Shriver National Institute of Child Health and Human Development, National Institutes of Health, Bethesda, Maryland

AMELIA P. BAILEY, MD
Director of Minimally Invasive Surgery, Fertility Associates of Memphis, Memphis, Tennessee

G. WRIGHT BATES, MD
Professor and Director, Reproductive Endocrinology and Infertility, Department of Obstetrics and Gynecology, University of Alabama Birmingham, Birmingham, Alabama

PAUL R. BREZINA, MD, MBA
Assistant Clinical Professor of Reproductive Endocrinology and Infertility, Vanderbilt University School of Medicine, Nashville; Consulting Gynecologist, Department of Surgery, St. Jude Children's Research Hospital; Director of Reproductive Genetics, Fertility Associates of Memphis, Memphis, Tennessee

NATALIE M. CRAWFORD, MD
Reproductive Endocrinology and Infertility, University of North Carolina, Chapel Hill, North Carolina

JIANCHI DING, PhD
Director, In Vitro Fertilization Laboratory, Fertility Associates of Memphis, Memphis, Tennessee

LAURA C. ECKLUND, MD
Obstetrics and Gynecology Resident, Carolinas Medical Center, Charlotte, North Carolina

RAYMOND W. KE, MD
Assistant Clinical Professor of Reproductive Endocrinology and Infertility, Vanderbilt University School of Medicine, Nashville; Consulting Gynecologist, Department of Surgery, St. Jude Children's Research Hospital; Director, In Vitro Fertilization Program, Fertility Associates of Memphis, Memphis, Tennessee

JAMES L. KLOSKY, PhD
Associate Member; Director of Psychological Services, Cancer Survivorship, St. Jude Children's Research Hospital, Memphis, Tennessee

PINAR H. KODAMAN, MD, PhD
Assistant Professor, Department of Obstetrics, Gynecology, and Reproductive Sciences, Yale University School of Medicine, New Haven, Connecticut

ERTUG KOVANCI, MD
Division of Reproductive Endocrinology and Infertility, Department of Obstetrics and Gynecology, Baylor College of Medicine, Houston, Texas

MIRIAM S. KRAUSE, MD
Physician, Fertility and Endocrine Associates, Louisville, Kentucky

WILLIAM H. KUTTEH, MD, PhD
Clinical Professor of Reproductive Endocrinology and Infertility, Vanderbilt University School of Medicine, Nashville; Consulting Gynecologist, Department of Surgery, St. Jude Children's Research Hospital; Director, Fertility Associates of Memphis, Memphis, Tennessee

RUTH LATHI, MD, FACOG
Associate Professor; Director of Recurrent Pregnancy Loss Program, Division of Reproductive Endocrinology and Infertility, Stanford University School of Medicine, Stanford, California

PAUL B. MARSHBURN, MD
Director, Reproductive Endocrinology and Infertility; Professor, Department of Obstetrics and Gynecology, Carolinas Medical Center, Carolinas Healthcare System, Charlotte, North Carolina

MICHELLE L. MATTHEWS, MD
Professor, Obstetrics and Gynecology; Director, 4th Year Medical Student Education; Associate Director, Reproductive Endocrinology, Carolinas Healthcare System, Charlotte, North Carolina

TOLGA B. MESEN, MD
Department of Obstetrics and Gynecology, University of North Carolina at Chapel Hill, Chapel Hill, North Carolina

STEVEN T. NAKAJIMA, MD
Clinical Professor and Co-Director, Clinical Operations, Stanford Fertility and Reproductive Medicine Center, Palo Alto, California

CARTER OWEN, MD
Program in Reproductive and Adult Endocrinology, Eunice Kennedy Shriver National Institute of Child Health and Human Development, National Institutes of Health, Bethesda, Maryland

AMY K. SCHUTT, MD
Division of Reproductive Endocrinology and Infertility, Department of Obstetrics and Gynecology, Baylor College of Medicine, Houston, Texas

LORA SHAHINE, MD, FACOG
Pacific North West Fertility and In Vitro Fertilization Specialists; Division of Reproductive Endocrinology and Infertility, Department of Obstetrics and Gynecology, University of Washington School of Medicine, Seattle, Washington

ANNE Z. STEINER, MD, MPH
Reproductive Endocrinology and Infertility, University of North Carolina, Chapel Hill, North Carolina

REBECCA S. USADI, MD
Reproductive Endocrinology and Infertility, Carolinas Medical Center, Charlotte, North Carolina

JOHANNA VON HOFE, MD
Department of Obstetrics and Gynecology, University of Alabama Birmingham, Birmingham, Alabama

STEVEN L. YOUNG, MD, PhD
Department of Obstetrics and Gynecology, University of North Carolina at Chapel Hill, Chapel Hill, North Carolina

Contents

> Educating couples about natural means to improve fertility should include a discussion about appropriate timing to initiate a diagnostic evaluation for infertility. Complete infertility testing for both male and female factors allows directed care for all abnormalities to optimize chances for conception.

> Oocyte number and quality decrease with advancing age. Thus, fecundity decreases as age increases, with a more rapid decline after the mid-30s. Patients more than 35 years old should receive prompt evaluation for causes of infertility after no more than 6 months of attempted conception. Patients with abnormal tests of ovarian reserve have a poorer prognosis and may need more expedited and aggressive treatment. Although oocyte donation is the best method to overcome age-related infertility, other treatment options may help women proceed quicker toward pregnancy. Patients at an advanced age should be counseled and evaluated before undergoing infertility treatments.

> Before initiating ovulation induction, it is important to evaluate the underlying cause of a patient's anovulation and to make lifestyle modifications or treat underlying medical conditions, as appropriate. Here, ovulation induction agents are discussed with attention to their pharmacology, indications for use, therapy regimens, and efficacy. Adjuvant therapies and appropriate monitoring are also reviewed.

> The desire to reproduce is one of the strongest human instincts. Many men and women in our society may experience situations that compromise their future fertility. The past several decades have seen an explosion of

technologies that have changed the historical limitations regarding fertility preservation. This review offers an overview of the state of the art within fertility preservation including surgical and medical interventions and therapies that necessitate the need for cryopreservation of eggs, sperm, and embryos. The review also addresses the psychological consequences of banking/not banking materials among patients in need of fertility preservation, particularly in the oncofertility context.

Management strategies for overweight and obese women with polycystic ovarian syndrome (PCOS) who desire fertility should include weight loss. Even a small reduction in body weight can improve ovulatory function and pregnancy rate and reduce adverse obstetric outcomes. New data suggest that letrozole should be considered as the new first-line medical treatment of anovulatory infertility in PCOS over clomiphene citrate. Second-line treatments for anovulatory infertility include in vitro fertilization, gonadotropins, or ovarian drilling.

Uterine leiomyoma, benign monoclonal tumors, afflict an estimated 60% of reproductive-aged women, with higher rates among African American women. Leiomyoma are associated with significant medical costs, impaired fertility potential, obstetric complications, and gynecologic morbidity. Currently, the effective clinical management of leiomyoma is limited by the fact that hysterectomy is the only cure. The purpose of this article is to provide the practitioner with a practical overview of the clinical management of this disease.

Endometriosis is a common gynecologic disorder that persists throughout the reproductive years. Although endometriosis is a surgical diagnosis, medical management with ovarian suppression remains the mainstay of long-term management with superimposed surgical intervention when needed. The goal of surgery should be excision or ablation of all visible disease to minimize risk of recurrence and need for repeat surgeries. When infertility is the presenting symptom, surgical therapy in addition to assisted reproductive technology can improve chances of conception; however, the treatment approach depends on stage of disease and other patient characteristics that affect fecundity.

Abnormal uterine bleeding is a common medical condition with several causes. The International Federation of Gynecology and Obstetrics published guidelines in 2011 to develop universally accepted nomenclature and a classification system. In addition, the American College of Obstetrics and Gynecology recently updated recommendations on evaluation of abnormal uterine bleeding and indications for endometrial biopsies. This article reviews both medical and surgical treatments, including meta-analysis reviews of the most effective treatment options.

Recurrent pregnancy loss (RPL) is a multifactorial condition. Approximately half of patients with RPL will have no explanation for their miscarriages. De novo chromosome abnormalities are common in sporadic and recurrent pregnancy loss. Testing for embryonic abnormalities can provide an explanation for the miscarriage in many cases and prognostic information. Regardless of the cause of RPL, patients should be reassured that the prognosis for live birth with an evidence-based approach is excellent for most patients. The authors review current evidence for the evaluation and treatment of RPL and explore the proposed use of newer technology for patients with RPL.

Progesterone production from the corpus luteum is critical for natural reproduction. Progesterone supplementation seems to be an important aspect of any assisted reproductive technology treatment. Luteal phase deficiency in natural cycles is a plausible cause of infertility and pregnancy loss, though there is no adequate diagnostic test. This article describes the normal luteal phase of the menstrual cycle, investigates the controversy surrounding luteal phase deficiency, and presents the current literature for progesterone supplementation during assisted reproductive technologies.

Premature ovarian failure is a devastating diagnosis for reproductive-aged women. The diagnosis is relatively easy. However, it has serious health consequences, including psychological distress, infertility, osteoporosis, autoimmune disorders, ischemic heart disease, and increased risk for mortality. Management should be initiated immediately to prevent long-term consequences. Hormone replacement therapy is the mainstay of management. Postmenopausal hormone replacement therapy studies should not be used to determine the risks of treatment in these young women.

This article focuses on the cause, pathophysiology, differential diagnosis of, and treatment options for vasomotor symptoms. In addition, it summarizes important points for health care providers caring for perimenopausal and postmenopausal women with regard to health maintenance, osteoporosis, cardiovascular disease, and vaginal atrophy. Treatment options for hot flashes with variable effectiveness include systemic hormone therapy (estrogen/progestogen), nonhormonal pharmacologic therapies (selective serotonin reuptake inhibitors, selective norepinephrine reuptake inhibitors, clonidine, gabapentin), and nonpharmacologic therapy options (behavioral changes, acupuncture). Risks and benefits as well as contraindications for hormone therapy are further discussed.

OBSTETRICS AND GYNECOLOGY CLINICS

FORTHCOMING ISSUES

June 2015
Best Practices in High-Risk Pregnancy
Lynn L. Simpson, *Editor*

September 2015
The Ob/Gyn Hospitalist
Jennifer Tessmer-Tuck and
Brigid McCue, *Editors*

December 2015
Contraception
Pamela S. Lotke and Bliss Kaneshiro,
Editors

RECENT ISSUES

December 2014
Infectious Diseases in Pregnancy
Geeta Swamy, *Editor*

September 2014
Pelvic Pain in Women
Mary McLennan, Andrew Steele, and
Fah Che Leong, *Editors*

June 2014
Substance Abuse During Pregnancy
Hilary Smith Connery and
William F. Rayburn, *Editors*

ISSUE OF RELATED INTEREST

Endocrinology Clinics of North America, December 2015 (Vol. 44)
Reproductive Endocrinology
Peter Lee and Christopher Houk, *Editors*

DOWNLOAD
Free App!

Review Articles
THE CLINICS

NOW AVAILABLE FOR YOUR iPhone and iPad

Foreword

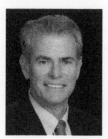

William F. Rayburn, MD, MBA
Consulting Editor

This issue of *Obstetrics and Gynecology Clinics of North America*, guest edited by Dr Michelle L. Matthews, provides an excellent update about reproductive endocrinology and infertility. The combined efforts of experts in this field highlight challenges to keep pace with a discipline that is advancing rapidly. Subjects in this issue were chosen with an emphasis on the needs and interests of practicing obstetrician-gynecologists. Discussions about common reproductive topics involve multidisciplinary approaches (leiomyoma, polycystic ovarian syndrome, abnormal uterine bleeding, endometriosis).

The issue also reflects the newest advances in infertility. For example, articles offer a focus on the newest advances in ovulation induction, cryopreservation of oocytes, preimplantation genetics, and emerging technologies with fertility preservation.

An effort was made to include tables and figures, which will aid readers to appreciate complex scientific concepts and improve understanding about such topics as progesterone and the luteal phase, premature ovarian failure, and nonhormonal treatment of vasomotor symptoms. The text contains references that have been limited mostly to published investigations in recent years.

The content of this update contains critical information that echoes the dynamic nature of reproductive endocrinology and infertility. The focus is on new and emerging diagnostics and techniques, presented from perspectives of balanced clinical values, ethics, and cost-effective care. Discussions about traditional practice are limited; instead, critical thinking is directed toward optimal and more contemporary care.

As advances unfold, obstetrician-gynecologists are urged to keep current with recent reports from the American Society of Reproductive Medicine, Society for Reproductive Investigation, and American College of Obstetricians and Gynecologists. Dr Matthews and her team of authors emphasize innovations in learning that apply

Obstet Gynecol Clin N Am 42 (2015) xiii–xiv
http://dx.doi.org/10.1016/j.ogc.2014.11.002
0889-8545/15/$ – see front matter © 2015 Published by Elsevier Inc.

obgyn.theclinics.com

directly to patient care. It is hoped that our readers will find this issue to be one of the most helpful and valuable resources in their daily practice.

William F. Rayburn, MD, MBA
Continuing Medical Education & Professional Development
MSC10 5580, 1 University of New Mexico
Albuquerque, NM 87131-0001, USA

E-mail address:
wrayburn@salud.unm.edu

Preface

Reproductive Endocrinology

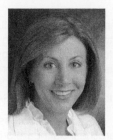

Michelle L. Matthews, MD
Editor

It is my honor to be the guest editor of this issue of *Obstetrics and Gynecology Clinics of North America*. This review of reproductive endocrinology focuses on recent updates to practice guidelines and current standards of care. Our goal is to provide clinicians with a logical and evidence-based approach to evaluation and management of common reproductive conditions.

We begin with a detailed review of the diagnostic evaluation of the infertile couple followed by a discussion of age-related infertility. A review of ovarian reserve testing and age-associated infertility is of importance to practitioners given the increasing percentage of women choosing to delay childbearing for personal or professional reasons. The following article presents an overview of recommendations for ovulation induction. The section concludes with a discussion of fertility preservation in the age of assisted reproduction. This is particularly timely given the recent change to American Society for Reproductive Medicine guidelines on oocyte cryopreservation.

Our review continues with a discussion of common reproductive concerns, including polycystic ovarian syndrome, leiomyomas, endometriosis, and abnormal uterine bleeding. An article on recurrent pregnancy loss is followed by a critical review of the ongoing debate regarding luteal phase insufficiency. The final section follows women as they advance through their reproductive years and includes a summary of premature ovarian failure and nonhormonal treatments for vasomotor symptoms.

I would like to express my gratitude to my fellow coauthors and colleagues who have provided their time and expertise to this publication. I hope that readers find it helpful in their clinical practice. I would also like to acknowledge the dedication of the individuals who performed the research, and the patients who participated in the research that is referenced in this issue.

In preparation of this review, I reflected on what changes occurred in reproductive endocrinology since completing my training in the late 1990s. At that time, we were not performing biopsies of embryos for genetic testing, cryopreserving oocytes, or successfully transplanting ovarian tissue. This year in particular marks the first report

Obstet Gynecol Clin N Am 42 (2015) xv–xvi
http://dx.doi.org/10.1016/j.ogc.2014.11.001
0889-8545/15/$ – see front matter © 2015 Elsevier Inc. All rights reserved.

of a birth after a complete uterine transplantation. It is really quite remarkable to consider what advances have occurred in a relatively short timeframe. It is difficult to predict where we will be in another decade, but I look forward to the future of reproductive medicine and the advances that will result in improved options and outcomes for our patients.

Michelle L. Matthews, MD
Professor of Obstetrics and Gynecology
Reproductive Endocrinology
Carolinas HealthCare System
1025 Morehead Medical Drive, Suite 500
Charlotte, NC 28204, USA

E-mail address:
Michelle.matthews@carolinashealthcare.org

Counseling and Diagnostic Evaluation for the Infertile Couple

Paul B. Marshburn, MD

KEYWORDS

- Infertility counseling • Optimizing natural fertility • Ovarian reserve testing
- Ovulatory dysfunction • Obstructive and nonobstructive male factor infertility
- Genetic causes of male factor infertility

KEY POINTS

- Proper counseling about the natural means to improve fertility should include a discussion about appropriate timing to initiate a diagnostic evaluation for infertility.
- Diagnostic evaluation of the infertile couple is best outlined by discussing the steps necessary for conception.
- Both male and female infertility factors should be investigated simultaneously to optimize all abnormalities for the best pregnancy outcomes.
- Coordination between gynecologists, reproductive endocrinologists, male reproductive urologists, and genetic counselors can be critical for conducting comprehensive diagnostic testing and determine safe and effective treatment options.

INTRODUCTION

Infertility is defined as a lack of pregnancy after 12 months of unprotected sexual intercourse with the same partner. The National Survey of Family Growth (NSFG) conducted by the Centers for Disease Control and Prevention indicates that, in the United States, the proportion of women aged 15 to 44 years who had ever accessed infertility care increased from 9% to 15% between 1982 and 1995, and then stabilized at 12% through 2010.[1,2] The upward trend in the rate for seeking infertility care most likely involves the decline in natural fertility with female age, an increased incidence of sexually transmitted infections, higher exposure to environmental toxins, and lifestyle factors such as smoking and obesity.

An estimated 75% of infertile couples will achieve conception after evaluation and treatment for infertility.[3] The success of therapeutic interventions depends on proper counseling and diagnostic evaluation of the infertile couple.

The author has nothing to disclose.
Department of Obstetrics and Gynecology, Carolinas Medical Center, Carolinas Healthcare System, P.O. Box 32861, Charlotte, NC 28232-2861, USA
E-mail address: Paul.Marshburn@carolinashelathcare.org

Obstet Gynecol Clin N Am 42 (2015) 1–14
http://dx.doi.org/10.1016/j.ogc.2014.10.001
0889-8545/15/$ – see front matter © 2015 Elsevier Inc. All rights reserved.

obgyn.theclinics.com

COUNSELING THE INFERTILE COUPLE

Initial counseling of infertile couples can naturally enhance their chance for conception and will dispel myths about unproven practices. Approximately 85% of couples should expect to become pregnant within 12 months of unprotected intercourse. Although the chance for pregnancy will be highest in the first 3 months, approximately 80% of couples destined to become pregnant within 1 year will achieve this goal by 6 months.[4] Women who are 35 to 40 years of age will have approximately one-half the cycle fecundity of women between 20 and 30 years of age.[5,6] Thus, earlier infertility evaluation is warranted after 6 months of unsuccessful efforts to conceive in women aged 35 years and older.[7] An infertility diagnostic evaluation does not need to be delayed in the presence of obvious menstrual irregularity, persistent sexual dysfunction, history of pelvic inflammatory disease, previous cancer chemotherapy, or male factor issues, including prior use of anabolic steroids or genital surgery.

NATURAL MEANS FOR ENHANCING CONCEPTION

The optimal frequency of intercourse during the fertile window is every 3 days or less and may begin 5 days before ovulation.[8] The male partner does not need to have ejaculatory abstinence for greater than 2 days in the periovulatory period, and in fact abstinence for greater than 5 days may adversely affect sperm quality.[9] In men with low sperm densities, daily ejaculation can actually increase sperm count.[10]

No evidence shows that the use of methods to predict ovulation increases the chance for conception in couples able to have regular intercourse. Ovulation predictor methods may produce false-positive and false-negative readings.[11] Of all the methods for ovulation detection, peak cervical mucus production predicts the fertile window more accurately than basal body temperature graphing, urinary luteinizing hormone (LH) monitoring, and use of a menstrual calendar.[12] If these methods are improperly performed or applied, they could actually impair fertility by causing couples to miss the timing for their fertile window.

Coital method or positioning for intercourse also has no apparent effect on conception rates. Women may remain supine or elevate their hips after intercourse to prevent the loss of semen from the vagina, but these practices have no benefit. Sperm can be found in the fallopian tubes within 15 minutes after intercourse around the time of ovulation.[13] Personal lubricants such as mineral oil, canola oil, or hydroxyethylcellulose-based lubricants have no known detrimental effect on sperm viability, whereas water-based lubricants such as K-Y or Astroglide have been shown to inhibit sperm motility in vitro.[14]

LIFESTYLE CONSIDERATIONS

Obesity is associated with ovulatory dysfunction, insulin resistance, and lower pregnancy rates after in vitro fertilization (IVF). Weight reduction of 10% to 15% of total body weight can improve ovulation rates and reduce the incidence of comorbid associations, such as hypertension and adult-onset diabetes mellitus, which as both risk factors for pregnancy complications. Women should be adequately supplementing their diet with 400 mcg of folate.[15] No specific dietary supplement for men or women has been proven to enhance fertility, but research remains active in this area.

Tobacco smoking has a detrimental impact on fertility and increases the risk of miscarriage.[16,17] Heavy use of alcohol should be avoided when attempting pregnancy, but an adverse effect of modest alcohol consumption (1 drink per day) on conception has not been proven. Caffeine consumption at the equivalent of 1 to 2 cups of coffee per day has no known negative effect on fertility when consumed by men or women.[18]

HISTORY AND PHYSICAL EXAMINATION OF THE WOMAN IN THE INFERTILE COUPLE

A discussion of the process of reproduction and conception will help the infertile couple understand the basis for diagnostic testing. A helpful construct is to discuss the infertility evaluation with regard to (1) ovarian factors, (2) abnormalities of the pelvic organ anatomy and function, and (3) the male factor. In at least one-third of couples, more than 1 potential cause for the infertility will be detected, and in approximately 20% of couples baseline testing will show no abnormality.

A preconception evaluation should include comprehensive medical, reproductive, and family history, along with discussion of genetic carrier screening. Secondary infertility should prompt careful attention to acquired conditions, including the outcome and complications of prior pregnancies, possible adhesions from interval pelvic surgery, endometriosis, and sexually transmitted infections. Records of prior infertility testing and treatment will help save time and resources. **Table 1** provides a summary of relevant historical points for assessing ovarian factors and abnormalities of the pelvic organ anatomy recommended by the American Society for Reproductive Medicine.[19]

THE EVALUATION OF OVARIAN FACTORS

An investigation for ovarian factors should include an evaluation of the regularity of ovulation and an assessment of ovarian reserve. Ovulatory dysfunction accounts for up to 40% of female factor infertility.[20] Obvious menstrual irregularity indicates a frequency of ovulation that would reduce fertility potential. Ovarian reserve refers to the number and quality of the oocytes that remain in the ovary. Oocyte quality refers to the capability of the egg to sustain normal fertilization and growth of that embryo for implantation and development into the birth of a viable offspring. In contrast to women with ovulatory dysfunction, those with diminished ovarian reserve (DOR) most often

---

Table 1
Summary of relevant history and physical examination findings for determining female factors in the infertile couple

History	Physical Examination
• Duration of infertility	• Weight, body mass index, blood pressure, and pulse
• Menstrual history	
• Pregnancy history	• Thyroid enlargement and presence of any nodules or tenderness
• Previous methods of contraception	
• Coital frequency and sexual dysfunction	• Breast secretions and their character
• Past surgery (procedures, indications)	• Signs of androgen excess
• Hospitalizations (illnesses or injuries)	• Vaginal or cervical abnormality or discharge
• Pelvic inflammatory disease (sexually transmitted diseases)	• Pelvic or abdominal tenderness, organ size, or masses
• Thyroid disease, galactorrhea, hirsutism	• Uterine size, shape, position, and mobility
• Abnormal pap smears or cervical surgeries	• Adnexal masses or tenderness
• Current medications and allergies	• Cul-de-sac masses, tenderness, or nodularity
• Family reproductive history	
• Exposure environmental hazards	
• Use of tobacco, alcohol, or illicit drugs	

Adapted from Practice Committee of the American Society for Reproductive Medicine. Diagnostic evaluation of the infertile female: a committee opinion. Fertil Steril 2012;98(2):302–7; with permission.

have regular menses unless the severity of DOR has progressed to the point of severe ovarian insufficiency.

Ovulatory Dysfunction

Infrequent ovulation is associated with an intermenstrual interval of less than 25 days or greater than 35 days, or a variation in the intermenstrual interval of greater than 5 days.[21] Premenstrual symptoms, referred to as *moliminal symptoms* (breast tenderness, irritability, mild headache), are typically associated with ovulatory cycles.

The only measure that proves ovulation has occurred is a positive pregnancy test after a conception cycle. Special diagnostic testing to confirm ovulation is not required in women with a history of regular cycles with premenstrual molimina. If an objective measure of ovulation is desired, a serum progesterone level can be obtained 7 days after a positive urinary LH determination. A concentration of progesterone of greater than 3 ng/mL is consistent with ovulation.[22]

When oligo-ovulation is present, a specific cause should be sought. The most common causes of ovulatory dysfunction include polycystic ovary syndrome, excessive psychological or physical stress, thyroid disorders, hyperprolactinemia, ovarian insufficiency, and medical conditions including obesity. Serum thyroid-stimulating hormone (TSH) and prolactin determinations will identify thyroid disorders and/or hyperprolactinemia. If hypothyroidism is suggested by an elevation of TSH along with an elevation in prolactin, levothyroxine replacement is indicated first to see if it will normalize an elevated prolactin level. Elevations of early follicular-phase follicle-stimulating hormone (FSH) levels greater than 10 mIU/mL are a threshold measure for DOR, whereas FSH levels of less than 4 mIU/mL may be encountered with hypothalamic oligo-ovulation.

Frequently no specific endocrine abnormality will be identified after the initial evaluation of women with ovulatory dysfunction. Most of the women with normal gonadotropin levels and no other known endocrine abnormality will be classified as having polycystic ovary syndrome (PCOS), exhibiting at least 2 of the 3 following characteristics: (1) hyperandrogenism (hirsutism, oily skin, acne), (2) irregular menses indicating oligo-ovulation, or (3) polycystic ovaries (>11 basal antral follicles, <10 mm in a single longitudinal image of each ovary by transvaginal ultrasound). This definition of PCOS, however, will also include some women with hypothalamic oligo-ovulation, because these women can exhibit PCOS-appearing ovaries with irregular menses. This distinction is important because the best method of ovulation induction will be different for these groups of women.

Ovarian Reserve

Testing to assess ovarian reserve includes early follicular phase FSH and estradiol levels, basal antral follicle (BAF) count measured with transvaginal ultrasound, and a serum anti-Müllerian hormone (AMH) level. For patient convenience, blood tests for ovarian reserve and ultrasound evaluation for BAF count can all be obtained in one visit on cycle day 2, 3, or 4 (with cycle day 1 the first day of full menstrual flow).

FSH and estradiol values should be correlated with the type of assay reported in the literature for levels indicating outcomes for normal ovarian reserve, diminished ovarian reserve, and ovarian insufficiency. Early follicular-phase levels of FSH levels are the most variable measure of ovarian reserve and should be obtained along with an estradiol level. An elevation in estradiol greater than 60 pg/mL with a normal range of FSH (<10 mIU/mL) is associated with both a poorer ovarian response during ovulation induction and a lower pregnancy rate with treatment.[23] The BAF count is measured as the sum of antral follicles in both ovaries less than 10 mm, as observed with transvaginal ultrasonography during the early follicular phase. An average BAF count in reproductive aged women is approximately 15. A BAF count of less than 10 has been correlated with poor ovarian response to ovulation induction stimulation and low chances for conception in that treatment cycle.[24] AMH is a protein secreted by granulosa cells and is an indirect measure of egg number and quality. AMH may be obtained during any phase of the menstrual cycle and is a more consistent measure of ovarian reserve.[25] Obesity and oral contraceptive pill use will suppress AMH levels. An AMH level of less than 1 ng/mL is associated with reduced ovarian response and chance for pregnancy in cycles of IVF.[26]

Ovarian reserve testing can be recommended for all women in the initial diagnostic evaluation of infertility, but is especially important for women who are older than 35 years, or have a history of ovarian surgery, chemotherapy or pelvic radiation, or unexplained infertility, or a family history of early menopause.[27] The finding of DOR does not indicate that a patient will not conceive, but rather has its greatest value in predicting the ovarian response to gonadotropin stimulation and chances for pregnancy with IVF.[28] Oocyte quality is more difficult to ascertain through ovarian reserve testing, but AMH levels seem to have the best predictive value for this measure of fertility potential.[29]

UTERINE AND PERITONEAL ABNORMALITIES AND INFERTILITY

The evaluation of uterine, tubal, and peritoneal factors is necessary to assess the likelihood of a favorable environment for gamete transport, fertilization, embryo implantation, and continued development of a pregnancy. Diagnostic procedures for evaluating the anatomy of the uterus, fallopian tubes, and peritoneal cavity provide different and complementary information. Hysterosalpingography remains the most versatile initial test for uterine cavity conformation, assessment of tubal patency, and evaluation of developmental abnormalities, such as a unicornuate, septate, or bicornuate uterus. Fluoroscopic or hysteroscopic selective tubal cannulation can confirm or exclude pathologic conditions causing proximal tubal occlusion determined on hysterosalpingography. This method uses an intrauterine catheter to selectively cannulate a fallopian tube and infuse dye or contrast to assess tubal patency or define intratubal disease.[30] Saline instillation sonography is superior to hysterosalpingography for evaluating endometrial polyps, submucosal fibroids, and adenomyosis.[31] Because of its increased expense and invasiveness, hysteroscopy is reserved for patients who require corrective intrauterine surgery.[32] The scheduling of hysteroscopy together with laparoscopy is an efficient way to evaluate and treat women with both intrauterine and peritoneal abnormalities. Laparoscopy is reserved for infertile women whose history, physical examination, and testing reveal the presence of certain adnexal masses, pelvic pain, or tubal abnormalities. With direct visualization of the peritoneal cavity, endometriosis and pelvic adhesions can be diagnosed and possibly corrected.

Table 2 summarizes the methods for assessing uterine, fallopian tube, and peritoneal abnormalities in women of the infertile couple, and outlines the relative advantages and disadvantages of each.

MALE REPRODUCTIVE HISTORY AND PHYSICAL EXAMINATION

A male factor contributes to infertility in up to 40% of couples.[33] Although the semen analysis remains the cornerstone for the initial male evaluation, other historical factors are important even when the semen analysis is normal. The approach for evaluating men with primary infertility (never having fathered a pregnancy) is the same as for men

Table 2 Methods for assessing uterine, fallopian tube, and peritoneal abnormalities in women with infertility					
	Uterine Cavity	Tubal Patency	Peritoneal Cavity	Advantages	Disadvantages
Hysterosalpingogram	+++	+++	+	Defines size and shape of uterine cavity, detects Müllerian and intratubal anomalies, profertility effect	Cannot assess size or depth of uterine tumors, no tubo-ovarian proximity evaluation
Saline instillation Sonography	++++	+	−	Excellent judge of cavity conformation, size and depth of uterine tumors Simple office procedure with lower cost and less pain Can view ovaries for BAF count, cysts	May assess tubal patency by seeing pelvic fluid but not tubal anatomy, no tubo-ovarian proximity evaluation, poor for severe intrauterine adhesions
Hysteroscopy	++++	−	−	Gold standard for uterine cavity evaluation Corrective surgery possible Adjunctive procedures with laparoscopy	Expensive, more invasive, more intensive instrumentation Unable to evaluate tubal anatomy
Laparoscopy	−	++++	++++	Best to identify and correct uterotubal, ovarian and peritoneal factors Tubal patency can be assessed	Expensive, more invasive, more intensive instrumentation Unable to evaluate intrauterine anatomy

with secondary infertility. The infertile man may present with underlying medical conditions that secondarily result in an abnormal semen analysis. Failure to evaluate for conditions such as testicular cancer and pituitary tumors that are associated with male factor infertility can have serious health consequences if not detected and treated.[34]

For most gynecologists and reproductive endocrinologists, a careful history and semen analysis will help direct a referral to an urologist with specialty training in male reproductive medicine for further physical examination. **Table 3** provides a summary of relevant historical points for assessing male factors contributing to infertility recommended by the American Society for Reproductive Medicine.[35]

SEMEN ANALYSIS

Semen analysis is the essential initial test for male fertility potential. Unless a man has a history of reduced libido, erectile dysfunction, premature ejaculation, hypospadias, and/or the inability to achieve intravaginal ejaculation, the finding of normal semen parameters would prompt no need for further male diagnostic evaluation. Even with no other remarkable historical risk factors, however, a man with a normal semen analysis could still have abnormal sperm function. In couples undertaking in vitro fertilization, normal semen parameters may still be associated with poor fertilization and/or abnormal embryo growth. At least 2 semen analyses are recommended because of the known variability in the total number of motile sperm cells among specimens. An abnormal finding on semen analysis may also represent a problem with collection or lack of prompt analysis after collection (within 30 minutes).[36]

Assessment of semen and sperm characteristics should be performed in a laboratory with technicians certified by proficiency testing according to the guidelines of the Clinical Laboratory Improvement Amendments.[37] Semen collection is preferably performed via masturbation at the andrology laboratory after 2 to 3 days of ejaculatory abstinence. **Table 4** provides the lower limits of the accepted World Health Organization reference values for semen analysis.[38]

The significance of a single semen parameter must be evaluated with regard to the other semen and sperm characteristics. Retrograde ejaculation should be suspected

---

Table 3
Summary of relevant history and physical examination findings for determining male factors in the infertile couple

History	Physical Examination
• A history of prior fertility • Coital frequency and timing • Duration of infertility and prior fertility • Childhood illnesses • Developmental history • Systemic medical illnesses (eg, diabetes mellitus and upper respiratory diseases) • Previous surgery • Medications • Sexual history (including sexually transmitted infections) • Exposures to gonadal toxins (including environmental and chemical toxins and heat)	• Examination of the penis, noting the location of the urethral meatus • Palpation and measurement of the testes • Presence and consistency of both the vasa and epididymides • Presence or absence of a varicocele • Body habitus • Hair distribution • Breast development

Adapted from Practice Committee of the American Society for Reproductive Medicine. Diagnostic evaluation of the infertile male: a committee opinion. Fertil Steril 2012;98(2):294–301; with permission.

Table 4 Lower limits of the accepted World Health Organization reference values for semen analysis	
Semen Parameter	Reference Value
Ejaculate volume	1.5 mL
pH	7.2
Sperm concentration	15×10^6 spermatozoa/mL
Total sperm number	39×10^6 spermatozoa/ejaculate
Percent motility	40%
Forward progression	32%
Normal morphology (Kruger strict)	4% normal
Sperm agglutination	Absent
Viscosity	≤ 2 cm thread after liquefaction

in a man with low semen volume and a history of genital surgery, retroperitoneal lymph node dissection, or diseases that impair the autonomic nervous system, such as diabetes mellitus. In these cases, the patient should be asked to return for a repeat semen sample after emptying the bladder. Evaluation of the postejaculation urine may demonstrate the presence of sperm, confirming retrograde ejaculation.[39]

The most clinically useful determination of sperm morphology is provided by microscopically analyzing specially stained sperm to obtain a strict anatomic evaluation of the sperm head, neck, and tail.[39] Strict morphologic sperm reports of less than 4% normal forms are associated with lower oocyte fertilization in vitro.[40] Careful proficiency testing of laboratory technicians is critical for accurate strict morphology assessment of sperm.

The finding of round cells in the microscopic assessment of semen indicates the presence of leukocytes, immature germ cells, or degenerating epithelial cells.[38] The use of peroxidase staining can help differentiate among these cell types. Peroxidase-positive cells are polymorphonuclear leukocytes and may represent genital tract infection or inflammation. Immature germ cells in semen may reveal a disorder in spermatogenesis.

The finding of very low numbers or absence of motile sperm cells in the ejaculate can be devastating to the infertile couple. **Table 5** includes a summary of the potential implications of abnormal semen analysis parameters. Many men with extremely depressed sperm counts can still achieve a conception, although assisted reproductive technology may be required.

MALE REPRODUCTIVE UROLOGY

Defining the cause of the male factor infertility is often best achieved in consultation with a urologist with training and expertise in male reproductive medicine. A reproductive urologist will examine the male genitalia and, if indicated, order hormonal and genetic laboratory testing. A low testicular volume (<15 mL) is a significant determinant for sperm production and indicates that the seminiferous tubules are either atrophic from lack of gonadotropin stimulation or atrophic because of a primary testicular process.

The physical examination by the male reproductive urologist can be assisted by ultrasonography of the male genital system. In the case of low semen volume (<1 mL) with no evidence of retrograde ejaculation, transrectal ultrasonography can reveal dilated seminal vesicles or ejaculatory ducts, suggesting partial or complete ductal

Table 5
Implications of abnormal semen parameters in the evaluation of male factor infertility

Parameter	Implication
Volume	• Low volume with decreased or absent sperm numbers: partial genital tract obstruction, androgen deficiency • Low volume with normal sperm concentration: problems with semen collection, partial retrograde ejaculation • High volume: possible genital tract infection
Sperm concentration	• Low numbers of sperm cells per milliliter: hypogonadism from hypothalamic/pituitary insufficiency or primary testicular dysfunction • Azoospermia (absent sperm): complete genital tract obstruction, primary testicular failure, complete hypothalamic/pituitary insufficiency, complete retrograde ejaculation
Motility	• Isolated severe low motility: toxins in seminal plasma or delayed analysis of specimen, prolonged period of ejaculatory abstinence • Low motility with global semen parameter abnormality: see causes listed previously for low or absent sperm concentration.
Morphology	• Total morphologic abnormality of a single type: possible rare genetic abnormality • Multiple abnormalities by strict morphology staining: most often unexplained
White or round cells	• Leukocytes: possible genital tract infection of inflammation • Immature sperm cells: possible disorder of spermatogenesis

obstruction.[41] Careful physical examination of the scrotum can identify a varicocele (enlarged testicular veins), absent vas deferens, firmness and pain of the epididymis, and testicular masses. Scrotal ultrasonography can help with ill-defined abnormalities detected through scrotal palpation, including small varicoceles, small testes located in the upper scrotum (cryptorchid), or testicular neoplasm that could be cancer.

A hormonal evaluation should be performed in men with oligozoospermia (sperm count <10 million/mL), diminished libido, erectile dysfunction, or phenotypic characteristics of endocrinopathy or genetic abnormality. An initial evaluation should include a measurement of serum FSH, LH, and testosterone. For men exhibiting a low serum testosterone level (<300 ng/mL), another level should be obtained along with a prolactin measurement. Some men with abnormal spermatogenesis have a normal serum FSH level, but an elevated serum FSH concentration (>14 mIU/mL) indicates primary testicular insufficiency, whereas a depressed FSH level (<4 mIU/mL) indicates hypogonadism from low gonadotropin production caused by pituitary or hypothalamic dysfunction.

Azoospermia (no sperm) or severe oligoasthenozoospermia (sperm count <5 million/mL) may be divided into one of the following diagnostic categories: (1) genital tract obstruction, (2) hypogonadotropic, nonobstructive azoospermia/oligoasthenozoospermia, or (3) testicular insufficiency, nonobstructive azoospermia/oligoasthenozoospermia. The diagnosis of azoospermia may be determined only after a semen specimen is centrifuged at 300 g for 15 minutes, with microscopic examination of the pellet. Identifying even a few spermatozoa in the ejaculate is useful because it indicates a higher rate of success with testicular sperm extraction (TESE) for IVF plus intracytoplasmic sperm injection (ICSI).[42] **Table 6** provides a reference for counseling men with severe azoospermia/oligoasthenozoospermia.

Table 6
Diagnostic evaluation for men with obstructive and nonobstructive azoospermia or severe oligoasthenozoospermia

Category	Physical Findings	Hormonal Evaluation	Other Testing
Obstructive	Possible congenital bilateral absence of the vas deferens, congenital or acquired obstructive stone or stricture of excurrent ductal system, normal testicular size	T: normal LH: normal FSH: normal	Dilated seminal vesicles on transrectal ultrasonography; postejaculatory urine analysis if absent semen on ejaculation; cystic fibrosis carrier screening
Nonobstructive: testicular insufficiency	Small testicular size, possible male eunuchoid habitus	T: low or normal LH: normal FSH: elevated	Karyotype, azoospermia factor microdeletion testing (AZF a, b, and c)
Nonobstructive: hypogonadotropic	Small testicular size, possible male eunuchoid habitus	T: low LH: low FSH: low	Possible brain MRI for lesion or tumor; gonadotropin replacement

Abbreviations: MRI, magnetic resonance imaging; T, testosterone.

GENETIC SCREENING OF MEN WITH MALE FACTOR INFERTILITY

Men with nonobstructive azoospermia or severe oligozoospermia have a higher risk of genetic abnormalities than fertile men.[43] Genetic abnormalities that result in aberrant spermatogenesis may be detected through karyotype and special testing for Y-chromosome microdeletions. Approximately 10% to 15% of men with nonobstructive azoospermia and 5% with severe oligozoospermia will have chromosomal abnormalities.[44,45] More than 50% of men with nonobstructive azoospermia/oligozoospermia who demonstrate structural or numerical chromosomal abnormalities will be found to have a karyotype of 46, XXY or Klinefelter syndrome.[46]

Specific microdeletions of the long arm of the Y chromosome are associated with azoospermia or severe oligozoospermia. Three regions on the Y chromosome have been named the azoospermia factor (AZF) regions: AZFa, AZFb, and AZFc. Men with the AZFc deletion are more likely to have sperm in their ejaculate and have a much higher chance of sperm retrieval via TESE. Very poor results are obtained from TESE in men with AZFa and AZFb deletions.[47,48] A convenient way to remember the most favorable prognosis for men with AZFc deletions is: AZF"a" is awful, AZF"b" is bad, and AZF"c" has conception. Couples should be counseled that sons of men with Y-chromosome microdeletions will inherit this chromosome and are very likely to have severe male factor infertility.[49]

Obstructive azoospermia from congenital bilateral absence of the vas deferens (CBAVD) is associated with a high risk of cystic fibrosis carrier status in affected men.[50] It is imperative, therefore, to test the female partner of a man affected by CBAVD. The safest measure is to sequence the cystic fibrosis gene in the female partner because some of the less common mutations may be missed on routine testing for cystic fibrosis carrier status.

All couples with severe male factor and either chromosomal or Y chromosomal microdeletions should receive genetic counseling to discuss prognostic information for offspring and choice of treatment options. With the advent of IVF and preimplantation genetic screening, the transfer of a single euploid embryo could be of great benefit to men with severe male factor infertility and structural or numerical chromosomal abnormalities.

SPECIALIZED CLINICAL TESTS OF SPERM FUNCTION

The availability of ICSI has greatly reduced the utility of testing for sperm–cervical mucous interaction and the acrosome reaction, and assays to determine sperm/oocyte penetration. Antisperm antibodies (ASA) may impair sperm motility, prevent the penetration of cervical mucous, and prevent oocyte fertilization.[51] The greatest utility for ASA testing is before IVF to determine whether direct sperm injection via ICSI is indicated.[52] A direct immunobead test is recommended, because it determines whether ASA are bound directly to the spermatozoa.

Future investigation may ultimately reveal clinically relevant testing of sperm function that improves the management of infertile couples. Men with abnormally high sperm DNA fragmentation have lower pregnancy rates after intrauterine insemination or IVF and ICSI.[53] Unfortunately, no treatment for abnormal DNA integrity has yet shown benefit, and the prognostic value of DNA integrity testing has not been clinically proven.[54] Excessive reactive oxygen species levels in semen generated by leukocytes and senescent sperm cells are correlated with sperm membrane damage and male factor infertility.[55] The development of a clinically practical test for excessive reactive oxygen levels in semen could allow for targeted treatment, such as shortening the period of ejaculatory abstinence before insemination or treatment with reducing vitamins such as vitamins E and C.[56]

THE CASE OF UNEXPLAINED INFERTILITY

How should infertile couples be counseled when the results of their diagnostic evaluation are all normal? This potentially frustrating circumstance can be approached by explaining the practical limitations of diagnostic testing. A more accurate description of their condition would be a status of having "underdiagnosed" infertility. The most likely factors contributing to unexplained infertility are issues relating to reduced sperm and egg quality, fertilization, or occult abnormalities of the fallopian tubes and the peritoneal cavity not diagnosed by hysterosalpingography or laparoscopy. The utility of IVF to diagnose problems with fertilization, sperm and egg quality, and embryo growth is obviously not practical. In this situation of unexplained infertility, the chance for pregnancy per menstrual cycle with continued natural attempts for pregnancy will be approximately 4% per cycle,[57] and this chance decreases with increased periods of infertility before evaluation and with the age of the female partner.[58] Couples with unexplained infertility can be reassured that they will have increased pregnancy rates with empiric ovulation induction and intrauterine insemination followed by IVF if necessary.[59]

REFERENCES

1. Chandra A, Stephen EH. Impaired fecundity in the United States: 1982–1995. Fam Plann Perspect 1998;30(1):34–42.
2. Chandra A, Copen CE, Stephen EH. Infertility and impaired fecundity in the United States, 1982–2010: data from the National Survey of Family Growth. Natl Health Stat Report 2014;67:1–18.
3. Chandra A, Copen CE, Stephen EH. Infertility service use in the United States: data from the National Survey of Family Growth, 1982–2010. Natl Health Stat Report 2014;73:1–20.

4. Gnoth C, Godehardt D, Godehardt E, et al. Time to pregnancy: results of the German prospective study and impact on the management of infertility. Hum Reprod 2003;18:1959–66.
5. Howe G, Westhoff C, Vessey M, et al. Effects of age, cigarette smoking, and other factors on fertility: findings in a large prospective study. BMJ 1985;290:1697–700.
6. Dunson DB, Baird DD, Colombo B. Increased infertility with age in men and women. Am J Obstet Gynecol 2004;103:51–6.
7. Zinaman MJ, Clegg ED, Brown CC, et al. Estimates of human fertility and pregnancy loss. Fertil Steril 1996;65:503–9.
8. Wilcox AJ, Dunson DB, Weinberg CR, et al. Likelihood of conception with a single act of intercourse: providing benchmark rates for assessment of post-coital contraceptives. Contraception 2001;63:211–5.
9. Elzanaty S, Malm J, Giwercman A. Duration of sexual abstinence: epididymal and accessory sex gland secretions and their relationship to sperm motility. Hum Reprod 2005;20:221–5.
10. Levitas E, Lunenfeld E, Weiss N, et al. Relationship between the duration of sexual abstinence and semen quality: analysis of 9,489 semen samples. Fertil Steril 2005;83:1680–6.
11. Practice Committee of American Society for Reproductive Medicine in collaboration with Society for Reproductive Endocrinology and Infertility. Optimizing natural fertility. Fertil Steril 2008;90:S1–6.
12. Stanford JB, Smith KR, Dunson DB. Vulvar mucus observations and the probability of pregnancy. Obstet Gynecol 2003;101:1285–93.
13. Settlage DS, Motoshima M, Tredway DR. Sperm transport from the external cervical as to the fallopian tubes in women: a time and quantitation study. Fertil Steril 1973;24:655–61.
14. Kutteh WH, Chao CH, Ritter JO, et al. Vaginal lubricants for the infertile couple: effect on sperm activity. Int J Fertil Menopausal Stud 1996;41:400–4.
15. Lumley J, Watson L, Watson M, et al. Periconceptional supplementation with folate and/or multivitamins for preventing neural tube defects. Cochrane Database Syst Rev 2001;(3):CD001056.
16. Winter E, Wang J, Davies MJ, et al. Early pregnancy loss following assisted reproductive technology treatment. Hum Reprod 2002;17:3220–3.
17. Ness RB, Grisso JA, Hirschinger N, et al. Cocaine and tobacco use and the risk of spontaneous abortion. N Engl J Med 1999;340:333–9.
18. Povey AC, Clyma JA, McNamee R, et al, Participating centres of CHAPS-UK. Modifiable and non-modifiable risk factors for poor semen quality: a case-referent study. Hum Reprod 2012;27:2799–806.
19. Practice Committee of the American Society for Reproductive Medicine. Diagnostic evaluation of the infertile female: a committee opinion. Fertil Steril 2012; 98(2):302–7.
20. Mosher WD, Pratt WF. Fecundity and infertility in the United States: incidence and trends. Fertil Steril 1991;56:192–3.
21. McCarthy JJ, Rockette HE. Prediction of ovulation with basal body temperature. J Reprod Med 1986;31:742–7.
22. Wathen NC, Perry L, Lilford RJ, et al. Interpretation of single progesterone measurement in diagnosis of anovulation and defective luteal phase: observations on analysis of the normal range. Br Med J (Clin Res Ed) 1984;288:7–9.
23. Licciardi FL, Liu HC, Rosenwaks Z, et al. Day 3 estradiol serum concentrations as prognosticators of ovarian stimulation response and pregnancy outcome in patients undergoing in vitro fertilization. Fertil Steril 1995;64:991–4.

24. Hendriks DJ, Mol BW, Bancsi LF, et al. Antral follicle count in the prediction of poor ovarian response and pregnancy after in vitro fertilization: a meta-analysis and comparison with basal follicle-stimulating hormone level. Fertil Steril 2005; 83:291–301.

25. Tsepelidis S, Devreker F, Demeestere I, et al. Stable serum levels of anti-Müllerian hormone during the menstrual cycle: a prospective study in normo-ovulatory women. Hum Reprod 2007;22:1837–40.

26. Muttukrishna S, McGarrigle H, Wakim R, et al. Antral follicle count, anti-Müllerian hormone and inhibin B: predictors of ovarian response in assisted reproductive technology? BJOG 2005;112:1384–90.

27. Sharara FI, Scott RT, Seifer DB, et al. The detection of diminished ovarian reserve in infertile women. Am J Obstet Gynecol 1998;179:804–12.

28. Broekmans FJ, Kwee J, Hendriks DJ, et al. A systematic review of tests predicting ovarian reserve and IVF outcome. Hum Reprod Update 2006;12:685–718.

29. Ebner T, Sommergruber M, Moser M, et al. Basal level of anti-Müllerian hormone is associated with oocyte quality in stimulated cycles. Hum Reprod 2006;21: 2022–6.

30. Valle RF. Tubal cannulation. Obstet Gynecol Clin North Am 1995;22:519–40.

31. Soares SR, Barbosa dos Reis MM, Camargos AF, et al. Diagnostic accuracy of sonohysterography, transvaginal sonography, and hysterosalpingography in patients with uterine cavity diseases. Fertil Steril 2000;73:406–11.

32. Hamilton JA, Larson AJ, Lower AM, et al. Routine use of saline hysterosonography in 500 consecutive, unselected, infertile women. Hum Reprod 1998;13:2463–73.

33. Thonneau P, Marchand S, Tallec A, et al. Incidence and main causes of infertility in a resident population (1,850,000) of three French regions (1988–1989). Hum Reprod 1991;6:811–6.

34. Honig SC, Lipshultz LI, Jarow J, et al. Significant medical pathology uncovered by a comprehensive male infertility evaluation. Fertil Steril 1994;62:1028–34.

35. Practice Committee of the American Society for Reproductive Medicine. Diagnostic evaluation of the infertile male: a committee opinion. Fertil Steril 2012; 98(2):294–301.

36. Guzick DS, Overstreet JW, Factor-Litvak P, et al. Sperm morphology, motility, and concentration in fertile and infertile men. N Engl J Med 2001;345:1388–93.

37. Clinical Laboratory Improvement Amendments (CLIA). Centers for Medicare & Medicaid Services Web site. 2014. Available at: http://www.cms.hhs.gov/CLIA/.

38. World Health Organization Department of Reproductive Health and Research. World Health Organization laboratory manual for the examination and processing of human semen. 5th edition. Geneva (Switzerland): World Health Organization; 2010.

39. Cooper TG, Noonan E, von Eckardstein S, et al. World Health Organization reference values for human semen characteristics. Hum Reprod Update 2010;16:231.

40. Kruger TF, Acosta AA, Simmons KF, et al. Predictive value of abnormal sperm morphology in in vitro fertilization. Fertil Steril 1988;49:112.

41. Jarow JP. Transrectal ultrasonography of infertile men. Fertil Steril 1993;60: 1035–9.

42. Bryson CF, Ramasamy R, Sheehan M, et al. Severe testicular atrophy does not affect the success of microdissection testicular sperm extraction. J Urol 2014; 191:175.

43. Foresta C, Garolla A, Bartoloni L, et al. Genetic abnormalities among severely oligospermic men who are candidates for intracytoplasmic sperm injection. J Clin Endocrinol Metab 2005;90:152–6.

44. Van Assche E, Bonduelle M, Tournaye H, et al. Cytogenetics of infertile men. Hum Reprod 1996;11:1–25.
45. Ravel C, Berthaut I, Bresson JL, et al. Prevalence of chromosomal abnormalities in phenotypically normal and fertile adult males: large-scale survey of over 10,000 sperm donor karyotypes. Hum Reprod 2006;21:1484–9.
46. De Braekeleer M, Dao TN. Cytogenetic studies in male infertility: a review. Hum Reprod 1991;6:245–50.
47. Oates RD, Silber S, Brown LG, et al. Clinical characterization of 42 oligospermic or azoospermic men with microdeletion of the AZFc region of the Y chromosome, and of 18 children conceived via ICSI. Hum Reprod 2002;17:2813–24.
48. Krausz C, Quintana-Murci L, McElreavey K, et al. Prognostic value of Y deletion analysis: what is the clinical prognostic value of Y chromosome microdeletion analysis? Hum Reprod 2000;15:1431–4.
49. Kent-First MG, Kol S, Muallem A, et al. The incidence and possible relevance of Y-linked microdeletions in babies born after intracytoplasmic sperm injection and their infertile fathers. Mol Hum Reprod 1996;2:943–50.
50. Anguiano A, Oates RD, Amos JA, et al. Congenital bilateral absence of the vas deferens. A primarily genital form of cystic fibrosis. JAMA 1992;267:1794–7.
51. Ayvaliotis B, Bronson R, Rosenfeld D, et al. Conception rates in couples where autoimmunity to sperm is detected. Fertil Steril 1985;43:739–42.
52. Check ML, Check JH, Katsoff D, et al. ICSI as an effective therapy for male factor with antisperm antibodies. Arch Androl 2000;45:125–30.
53. Collins JA, Barnhart KT, Schlegel PN, et al. Do sperm DNA integrity tests predict pregnancy with in vitro fertilization? Fertil Steril 2008;89:823–31.
54. Practice Committee of the American Society for Reproductive Medicine. The clinical utility of sperm DNA integrity testing. Fertil Steril 2008;90:S178–80.
55. Kim JG, Parthasarathy S. Oxidation and the spermatozoa. Semin Reprod Endocrinol 1998;16:235–9.
56. Marshburn PB, Giddings A, Causby S, et al. Influence of ejaculatory abstinence on seminal total antioxidant capacity and sperm membrane lipid peroxidation. Fertil Steril 2014;102:705–10.
57. Guzick DS, Sullivan MW, Adamson GD, et al. Efficacy of treatment for unexplained infertility. Fertil Steril 1998;70:207–13.
58. Collins JA, Burrows EA, Wilan AR. The prognosis for live birth among untreated infertile couples. Fertil Steril 1995;64:22–8.
59. Practice Committee of the American Society for Reproductive Medicine. Effectiveness and treatment for unexplained infertility. Fertil Steril 2006;86(4):S111–4.

Age-related Infertility

Natalie M. Crawford, MD*, Anne Z. Steiner, MD, MPH

KEYWORDS

- Aging • Infertility • Ovarian reserve • Advanced maternal age • Donor oocytes

KEY POINTS

- Fecundability decreases with increasing age.
- Evaluation for etiologies of infertility should be offered to women more than 35 years of age who have failed to conceive after 6 months.
- Abnormal tests for ovarian reserve should result in referral to an infertility specialist, as these patients need prompt evaluation and potentially more expedited and aggressive treatment.
- Oocyte donation provides the best chance for successful conception in patients with age-related infertility.
- Pregnancy at an advanced maternal age carries more risks for both mother and fetus, and patients should be fully informed and evaluated for potential complications before proceeding with infertility treatments.

INTRODUCTION

Societal shifts, triggered by a greater focus on education and careers, have resulted in a trend toward delayed childbearing in American women. Between 1970 and 2002, the percentage of first births in women more than 30 years of age increased 6-fold.[1–5] Along with the increase in maternal age has been an expansion in the number of women attempting to conceive at an age when the probability of conception (fecundability) is significantly decreased. The proportion of women who remain childless increases progressively with increased age at time of marriage: 6% at age 20 to 24 years, 9% at age 25 to 29 years, 15% at age 30 to 34 years, 30% at age 35 to 39 years, and 64% at ages more than 40 years.[6]

Although fertility declines with age of both men and women, the risk of infertility (ie, failure to achieve successful pregnancy after 12 months of attempt conception) has a stronger correlation with maternal age.[7] Historical studies have shown that fertility decreases at 32 years of age, with an increase in the rate of decline after 37 years of

Disclosure: The authors have nothing to disclose.
Reproductive Endocrinology and Infertility, University of North Carolina, 4001 Old Clinic Building, CB 7570, Chapel Hill, NC 27599, USA
* Corresponding author.
E-mail address: natalie_crawford@med.unc.edu

Obstet Gynecol Clin N Am 42 (2015) 15–25
http://dx.doi.org/10.1016/j.ogc.2014.09.005
0889-8545/15/$ – see front matter © 2015 Elsevier Inc. All rights reserved.

obgyn.theclinics.com

age.[7–9] A recent Danish study revealed peak fecundability at age 29 to 30 years in parous women and 27 to 28 years in nulliparous women. Furthermore, both the overall decrease in fecundability and the rate of decline in fecundability are greater in nulliparous women.[10]

The cause of age-related infertility is multifactorial. There is a demonstrated decrease in oocyte number as women progress through their reproductive years.[11,12] Furthermore, the rate of miscarriage and chromosomal abnormalities increases with increasing maternal age.[13] Aging is also associated with an increase in disorders that may impair fertility such as tubal disease, leiomyomas, and endometriosis.[14]

The impact of age-related behaviors, such as a decrease in sexual activity, on fertility is difficult to quantify. A French study of women with azoospermic husbands undergoing insemination revealed a decrease in pregnancy rates with increasing age. Cumulative pregnancy rates over 12 insemination cycles were 74% for women less than 31 years, 62% in women aged 31 to 35 years, and 54% in women more than 35 years of age.[15] However, a recent study showed that although timing of intercourse improved with age, both the frequency of intercourse and fecundability decreased with age.[10] This finding suggests that a decline in sexual behavior may contribute to, but is not the sole cause of, the decrease in fecundability seen with increasing age.

Reproductive aging is the natural process of declining fecundability as a woman progresses through the stages of puberty, fertility, the menopause transition, and menopause. However, the rate at which a woman moves through these stages can vary per individual.[16] Therefore, women of the same reproductive age can be at different stages in their reproductive lifespans. Because of this age-related decline in fertility, important consideration should be given to women planning or attempting to conceive in their later reproductive years. Current recommendations are to proceed with an evaluation for infertility after 6 months of attempted conception in a woman more than 35 years of age.[14]

DISCUSSION
Physiology of Reproductive Aging

Women are born with a finite number of oocytes. The peak in oocyte number occurs in utero, with 6 to 7 million oogonia at 16 to 20 weeks of gestation. From this point on, follicle number continues to decrease because of apoptosis of the nondominant follicles. At birth, 1 million to 2 million oocytes remain and only 300,000 to 500,000 are present when puberty begins. Follicle atresia increases at 37 years, when about 25,000 follicles remain. At the onset of menopause, fewer than 1000 follicles remain.[11,12,17]

The shrinking pool of oocytes results in decreased secretion of inhibin B from small preantral follicles. This loss of inhibition allows pituitary follicle-stimulating hormone (FSH) secretion to increase.[18,19] As FSH increases in the early follicular phase, aging ovaries show more rapid follicular development and an earlier selection of the dominant follicle.[20,21] This is clinically represented as a shorter follicular phase and irregular menstrual cycles, but these changes only become evident after significant ovarian aging has occurred.[22,23] Furthermore, the earlier increase in FSH level also frequently results in selection of more than 1 dominant follicle, explaining the increased rate of dizygotic twinning seen in natural conceptions at an advanced maternal age.[24]

The decrease in follicular number is coupled with a concurrent decrease in oocyte quality. An increased rate of chromosomal abnormalities and miscarriage has been shown with advancing maternal age (**Fig. 1**).[25–27] Studies suggest that most oocytes from women more than 40 years of age are chromosomally abnormal. The most

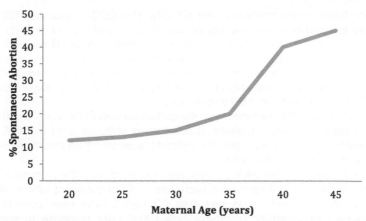

Fig. 1. Spontaneous abortions by maternal age. (*Data from* Hassold T, Chiu D. Maternal age-specific rates o numerical chromosomal abnormalities with specific reference to trisomy. Hum Genet 1985;70:11–17.)

common chromosomal abnormality seen with increasing age is trisomy.[27] The increase in aneuploidy in older oocytes is due to meiotic nondisjunction. A study evaluating oocytes from naturally cycling young women (20–25 years of age) and older women (40–45 years of age) revealed that 79% of the older oocytes had meiotic spindle abnormalities compared with 17% in the younger group.[28] Furthermore, the rate of significant chromosomal abnormalities in live births is 1 in 500 in women less than age 30 years, 1 in 80 at age 35 years, and 1 in 20 at age 45 years.[29]

Tests of Ovarian Reserve

Measures of ovarian reserve attempt to quantify a woman's reproductive potential by estimating the number of remaining oocytes. Ovarian reserve tests have been used along with menstrual history to estimate where a woman is in the process of reproductive aging. Measures of ovarian reserve predict oocyte yield following ovarian hyperstimulation and predict pregnancy following assisted reproductive technology (ART) in older women.[30] A small study suggests that measures of ovarian reserve may be predictors of natural fertility among women more than 30 years of age; however, definitive, larger studies are lacking.[31] Tests of ovarian reserve aid in counseling and selection of appropriate treatment of women with infertility.

- Early follicular phase FSH: A decrease in oocyte number results in decreased negative feedback from inhibin B and a resultant increase in FSH secretion in the early follicular phase.[18,21] An early follicular (cycle day 3) FSH cutoff value of greater than 10 IU/L has a high specificity (80%–100%) but lower sensitivity (10%–30%) for predicting poor ovarian response to stimulation.[18,21,32] FSH levels can be measured in serum or in urine.[33]
- Early follicular phase estradiol: Estradiol alone has limited utility in determining ovarian reserve. However, early follicular estradiol levels can aid in the interpretation of FSH values. With earlier selection of a dominant follicle, as seen with reproductive aging, estradiol levels increase in the early follicular phase and may suppress FSH secretion. Therefore, increased estradiol levels (>60–80 pg/mL) with normal FSH values (<10 IU/L) suggest diminished ovarian reserve. Women with increased FSH and estradiol levels are poor-prognosis patients for ART.[34,35]

- Clomiphene citrate challenge test (CCCT): The CCCT measures FSH levels before (cycle day 3) and after (cycle day 10) 5 days of stimulation with 100 mg of clomiphene citrate (cycle days 5–9). A decrease in inhibin B secretion from a small cohort of follicles provides less negative feedback on clomiphene-induced pituitary hormone release, resulting in an increased cycle day 10 FSH value.[36] The CCCT has higher sensitivity (13%–66%) but lower specificity (67%–100%) than basal FSH values alone.[37]
- Inhibin B: Inhibin B is secreted from the granulosa cells of the small antral follicles in the follicular phase. However, it has limited utility as a measure of ovarian reserve because it varies widely throughout the cycle[38,39] and must be measured during the early follicular phase.
- Antimullerian hormone (AMH): AMH, also secreted from the granulosa cells or preantral follicles, is important in recruitment of the dominant follicle. AMH declines with age, and values less than 0.7 ng/mL have been correlated with decreased fecundability in natural cycles and poor response to stimulation with ART.[30,40,41] AMH is unaffected by cycle day.[42] Cutoff values between 0.2 and 0.7 ng/mL have a sensitivity of 40% to 97% and a specificity of 78% to 92% in predicting poor response to ovarian stimulation.[29]
- Antral follicle count (AFC): AFC is the determination of all follicles with a mean diameter 2 to 10 mm by transvaginal ultrasonography in the early follicular phase. Histologic studies have correlated AFC with number of remaining primordial follicles.[43] A low AFC, less than 3 to 10 total follicles, has been associated with decreased success in achieving pregnancy following ART.[44] An AFC of fewer than 3 to 4 follicles has a sensitivity of 9% to 73% and a specificity of 73% to 100% for predicting poor response to ovarian stimulation.[29] Thus, AFC is best suited to help predict a patient who may have a poor response to stimulation with ART.

Management and Treatment

When using tests of ovarian reserve to determine a woman's reproductive potential, results should be compared with that of a woman her own age.[45] However, absolute cutoff values should be used when predicting ovarian response to stimulation. For example, an AMH level of 1.0 ng/mL in a 30-year-old woman suggests low ovarian reserve for her age. However, that patient would be unlikely to have poor oocyte yield (<4 oocytes) in response to controlled ovarian hyperstimulation. Therefore, tests of ovarian reserve should be interpreted with caution, because abnormal results do not define sterility, especially among young women. The predictive value of such tests appears to depend on the woman's age. However, an abnormal test indicates a need for a prompt evaluation and potentially a more aggressive approach in management.

There is no specific treatment of diminished ovarian reserve. The only treatment option to overcome age-related infertility is in vitro fertilization (IVF) with donor oocytes. Note that measures of ovarian reserve do not predict oocyte quality. A woman's risk of having a fetus affected by aneuploidy is driven by maternal age not ovarian reserve.[46]

Patients seeking pregnancy at an older age, patients more than 35 years of age without conception after 6 months of unprotected intercourse, or patients with diminished ovarian reserve should all be seen by an infertility specialist. In general, an infertility evaluation includes determination of ovulatory status, tests of ovarian reserve, evaluation of tubal and uterine anatomy, and semen analysis. If these tests return normal, then empirical treatment is usually undertaken with controlled ovarian hyperstimulation, intrauterine insemination, or in vitro fertilization. However, these options are often limited by the woman's age-related potential for reproduction.

The mean age of all patients undergoing IVF is 36 years.[47] Sixty-four percent of all IVF cycles are in women aged 30 to 39 years, with 24% of cycles in women aged 40 years and older.[47] The live birth rate per IVF cycle is directly correlated with maternal age. Recent US Centers for Disease Control and Prevention data for all fresh, nondonor IVF cycles in 2011 reported a live birth rate of 40% in women less than 35 years of age. This rate decreases as women age: 32% at 35 to 37 years, 22% at 38 to 40 years, 12% at 41 to 42 years, 5% at 43 to 44 years, and less than 1% in women older than 44 years (**Fig. 2**).[47]

Even with IVF, the likelihood of successful ongoing pregnancy is compromised by age. After the age of 30 years, the probability for ongoing pregnancy decreases by about 1.5% per year.[48] The rate of implantation decreases by more than two-thirds after the age of 40 years, likely reflecting poor embryo quality.[49] Miscarriage rates after IVF cycles are 15% in women less than 35 years old, 25% in women at age 40 years, and more than 70% in women more than 44 years of age.[47] The likelihood of success with IVF decreases because of a diminished response to stimulation, a lower chance of proceeding to oocyte retrieval and embryo transfer, and both lower pregnancy rates and live birth rates per transfer.[47] Poor embryo quality and increasing aneuploidy rates with older oocytes cannot be overcome with IVF alone. Results of studies evaluating chromosomal screening before embryo transfer have shown that there is a decline in reproductive potential of embryos even after controlling for aneuploidy.[50]

The use of IVF with donor oocytes has expanded the reproductive options of many women, especially those with age-related infertility. Pregnancy success rates are much higher and miscarriage rates are lower than in age-matched controls. When using donor oocytes, the live birth rate per embryo transfer is 55% across all age groups.[47] An analysis of cycles from the Society of Assisted Reproductive Technology (SART) database revealed that age affects IVF outcomes with donor oocytes. The live birth rate in recipients less than the age of 35 years was 56%, whereas the live birth rate for recipients aged 45 to 49 years and greater than 50 years was 52% and

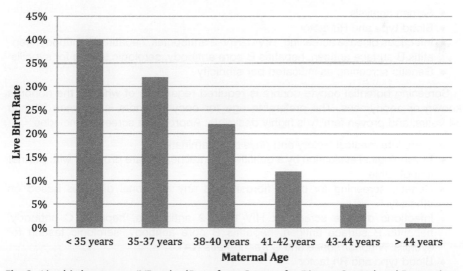

Fig. 2. Live birth rates per IVF cycle. (*Data from* Centers for Disease Control and Prevention, American Society for Reproductive Medicine Society for Assisted Reproductive Technology. 2011 assisted reproductive technology: national summary report. Atlanta (GA): Centers for Disease Control and Prevention; 2013.)

48%, respectively. However, the absolute live birth rates were still high.[51] The 2012 recommendations for gamete donation by the American Society for Reproductive Medicine (ASRM) provide current guidelines for screening oocyte donors and evaluation of the recipient. Indications for oocyte donation include[52]:

- Hypergonadotropic hypogonadism
- Advanced reproductive age
- Diminished ovarian reserve
- Genetic carriers
- Poor oocyte or embryo quality with previous failed IVF cycles

The recipient of the donor oocytes needs to be evaluated and screened before proceeding with the cycle. The increased risks for maternal complications in older women underscore the importance of this evaluation. Recommended screening includes[52]:

- Complete medical history and physical examination
- Psychological evaluation by a qualified mental health care provider, with partner if applicable
- Assessment of the uterine cavity, either with saline-infused sonography, hysterosalpingogram, or hysteroscopy
- Infectious disease screening: human immunodeficiency virus (HIV)-1/HIV-2 antibodies, hepatitis C antibody, hepatitis B surface antigen, hepatitis B core antibody, serologic testing for syphilis, *Neisseria gonorrhoeae* and *Chlamydia trachomatis* nucleic acid testing (NAT)
- Preconception screening: rubella and varicella titers, blood type and Rh factor, antibody screen
- If the recipient is more than the age of 45 years, further recommendations include a thorough medical evaluation with cardiovascular testing and referral to maternal fetal medicine to discuss risks with pregnancy at an advanced age

The partner of the recipient also requires evaluation with:

- Semen analysis
- Blood type and Rh factor
- Infectious disease screening: HIV-1/HIV-2 antibodies, hepatitis C antibody, hepatitis B surface antigen, hepatitis B core antibody, serologic testing for syphilis
- Genetic screening as indicated per ethnicity

Screening potential oocyte donors is required regardless of whether the donor is known or anonymous. The preferable age for oocyte donors is between 21 and 34 years, and proven fertility is highly desirable. Appropriate screening includes[52]:

- Complete medical history and physical examination
- Psychological evaluation by a qualified mental health care provider, with partner if applicable
- Genetic screening for cystic fibrosis and any additional diseases based on ethnicity
- Infectious disease screening: HIV-1/HIV-2 antibodies, hepatitis C antibody, hepatitis B surface antigen, hepatitis B core antibody, serologic testing for syphilis, *N gonorrhoeae* and *C trachomatis* NAT
- Blood type and Rh factor
- Verification of no recent tattoos or body piercings within the past 12 months

Furthermore, it is important to disclose all risks to the potential donor, including ovarian hyperstimulation syndrome (1%–2% of donor cycles), ovarian torsion, and risk of bleeding or infection with oocyte retrieval.[52] Data do not show an association between repetitive oocyte donation and future cancer development or diminished ovarian reserve. However, ASRM recommends limiting oocyte donation to 6 total cycles.[53]

Another potential option for patients of advancing age is the option for elective oocyte cryopreservation. The technique of oocyte vitrification has made oocyte cryopreservation for social reasons a possibility.[54,55] Although not a treatment of age-related infertility, oocyte cryopreservation is a preventative measure in attempt to conserve a woman's reproductive potential. Success rates after oocyte cryopreservation are based on data from oocyte donation programs. The live birth rates per 6 oocytes frozen at age 30 and 35 years are estimated at 24% and 18%, respectively.[56] Note that the effectiveness of oocyte cryopreservation for older or infertile women has not been proved.

Maternal and Fetal Risks

Pregnancy at an advanced maternal age has been correlated with an increased risk of specific adverse pregnancy outcomes. Advanced maternal age has been shown to be an independent risk factor for miscarriage, chromosomal abnormalities, congenital abnormalities, gestational diabetes, severe preeclampsia, placenta previa, and cesarean delivery. Furthermore, maternal age of 40 years or more was associated with a further increase in risk for placental abruption, preterm delivery, low birth weight, intrauterine growth restriction, stillbirth, and perinatal mortality.[57–60] One potential explanation for the increase in perinatal complications with advancing maternal age may be a failure of the uterine vasculature to adapt to the increased hemodynamic demand with pregnancy.[61] In addition, older patients are at an increased risk for multiple gestations, both in natural and assisted cycles, increasing the overall rate of perinatal complications. Pregnancy at an advanced maternal age is high risk, and antenatal testing during pregnancy is recommended.

It is difficult to draw conclusions about the impact that pregnancy with donor oocytes may have on maternal and fetal risks associated with advancing age. As previously discussed, the probability of live birth is 55% across all maternal ages with the use of donor oocytes.[47] Furthermore, the risk of miscarriage and chromosomal abnormalities is decreased in this population compared with women using their own oocytes.[62] However, the associations with preeclampsia, gestational diabetes, stillbirth, intrauterine growth restriction, and perinatal mortality likely persist because of impaired placentation and progressive uterine vascular endothelial damage with age.[57,59–62] Furthermore, oocyte donation in women of older age, especially women in their 50s, poses unique ethical issues. Therefore, ASRM has recommended that oocyte donation be discouraged when the recipient is more than the age of 50 years with any underlying medical problems or more than the age of 55 without such issues.[62]

SUMMARY

With the societal shift toward delayed childbearing, it is important for providers to remember that age is still the best marker for reproductive potential. However, patients of advancing age are capable of achieving pregnancy, especially in the era of advanced reproductive technology and donor oocytes. Pregnancy at an advanced maternal age has risks. Patients should be fully counseled and educated regarding options for conception and the implications of advancing age on both maternal and fetal outcomes.

REFERENCES

1. US Bureau of the Census. Percent of people 25 years and over who have completed high school or college, by race, Hispanic origin and sex: selected years 1940 to 2004 (noninstitutionalized population). 2005. Available at: http://www.census.gov/population/socdemo/education/tabA-2.pdf. Accessed December 29, 2006.
2. Stephen EH, Chandra A. Declining estimates of infertility in the United States: 1982-2002. Fertil Steril 2006;86:516–23.
3. Mathews TJ, Hamilton BE. Mean age of mother, 1970-2000. Natl Vital Stat Rep 2002;51:1–13.
4. Ventura SJ, Hamilton BE, Sutton PD. Revised birth and fertility rates for the United States, 2000 and 2001. Natl Vital Stat Rep 2003;51:1.
5. Martin JA, Hamilton BE, Ventura SJ, et al. Births: final data from 2000. Natl Vital Stat Rep 2002;50.
6. Menken J, Trussel J, Larsen U. Age and infertility. Science 1986;233:1389–94.
7. Practice Committee of the American Society for Reproductive Medicine. Definitions of infertility and recurrent pregnancy loss: a committee opinion. Fertil Steril 2013;99:63.
8. van Noord-Zaadstra BM, Looman CW, Alsbach H, et al. Delaying childbearing: effect of age on fecundity and outcome of pregnancy. Br Med J 1991;302: 1361–5.
9. Tietze C. Reproductive span and rate of reproduction among Hutterite women. Fertil Steril 1957;8:89–97.
10. Rothman KJ, Wise LA, Sorensen HT, et al. Volitional determinants and age-related decline in fecundability: a general population prospective cohort study in Denmark. Fertil Steril 2013;99:1958–64.
11. Baker TG. A quantitative and cytological study of germ cells in human ovaries. Proc R Soc Lond B Biol Sci 1963;158:417–33.
12. Block E. Quantitative and morphologic investigations of the follicular system in women; variations at different ages. Acta Anat (Basel) 1952;14:108–23.
13. Stein A. A woman's age, childbearing, and childrearing. Am J Epidemiol 1985; 121:327–42.
14. Practice Committee of the American Society for Reproductive Medicine. Female age related fertility decline. Fertil Steril 2014;101:633–4.
15. Schwartz D, Mayaux MJ. Female fecundity as a function of age: results of artificial insemination in 2193 nulliparous women with azoospermic husbands. Federation CECOS. N Engl J Med 1982;306:404–6.
16. Soules MR, Sherman S, Parrott E, et al. Executive summary: Stages of Reproductive Aging Workshop (STRAW). Fertil Steril 2001;76:874–8.
17. Faddy MJ, Gosden RG. A model conforming the decline in follicle numbers to the age of menopause in women. Hum Reprod 1992;7:1342–6.
18. Seifer DB, Scott RT, Bergh PA, et al. Women with declining ovarian reserve may demonstrate a decrease in serum inhibin B before a rise in day 3 follicle-stimulating hormone. Fertil Steril 1999;72:63–5.
19. Burger HG, Dudley EC, Hopper JL, et al. Prospectively measured levels of follicle-stimulating hormone, estradiol, and the dimeric inhibins during the menopausal transition in a population-based cohort of women. J Clin Endocrinol Metab 1999;84:4025–30.
20. de Koning CH, Popp-Snijiders C, Schoemaker J, et al. Elevated FSH concentrations in imminent ovarian failure are associated with higher FSH and LH pulse amplitude and response to GnRH. Hum Reprod 2000;15:1452–6.

21. Klein NA, Battaglia DE, Fujimoto VY, et al. Reproductive aging: accelerated ovarian follicular development associated with a monotropic follicle-stimulating hormone rise in normal older women. J Clin Endocrinol Metab 1996;81: 1038–45.
22. Klein NA, Harper AJ, Houmard BS, et al. Is the short follicular phase in older women secondary to advanced or accelerated dominant follicle development? J Clin Endocrinol Metab 2002;87:5746–50.
23. den Tonkelaar I, te Velde ER, Looman CW. Menstrual cycle length preceding menopause in relation to age at menopause. Maturitas 1998;29:115–23.
24. Beemsterboer SN, Homburg R, Gorter NA, et al. The paradox of declining fertility but increasing dizygotic twinning rates with advancing maternal age. Hum Reprod 2006;21:1531–2.
25. Smith K, Buyalos R. The profound impact of patient age on pregnancy outcome after early detection of fetal cardiac activity. Fertil Steril 1996;65:35–40.
26. Balasch J, Gratacos E. Delayed childbearing: effects on fertility and the outcome of pregnancy. Curr Opin Obstet Gynecol 2012;24:187–93.
27. Hassold T, Chiu D. Maternal age-specific rates o numerical chromosomal abnormalities with specific reference to trisomy. Hum Genet 1985;70:11–7.
28. Battaglia DE, Goodwin P, Klein NA, et al. Influence of maternal age on meiotic spindle assembly in oocytes from naturally cycling women. Hum Reprod 1996; 11:2217–22.
29. Hook E. Rates of chromosomal abnormalities at different maternal ages. Obstet Gynecol 1981;58:282.
30. Practice Committee of the American Society for Reproductive Medicine. Testing and interpreting measures of ovarian reserve: a committee opinion. Fertil Steril 2012;98:1407–15.
31. Steiner AZ, Herring AH, Kesner JS, et al. Antimullerian hormone as a predictor of natural fecundability in women aged 30-42 years. Obstet Gynecol 2011;117: 798–804.
32. Roberts JE, Spandorfer S, Fasouliotis SJ, et al. Taking a basal follicle-stimulating hormone history is essential before initiating in vitro fertilization. Fertil Steril 2005; 83:37–41.
33. Qiu Q, Kuo A, Todd H, et al. Enzyme immunoassay method for total urinary follicle-stimulating hormone (FSH) and its application for measurement of total urinary FSH. Fertil Steril 1998;69:278–85.
34. Licciardi FL, Liu HC, Rosenwaks Z. Day 3 estradiol serum concentrations as prognosticators of ovarian stimulation response and pregnancy outcome in patients undergoing in vitro fertilization. Fertil Steril 1995;64:991–4.
35. Buyalos RP, Daneshmand S, Brzechffa PR. Basal estradiol and follicle-stimulating hormone predict fecundity in women of advanced reproductive age undergoing ovulation induction therapy. Fertil Steril 1997;68:272–7.
36. Hofmann GE, Danforth DR, Seifer DB. Inhibin-B: the physiologic basis of the clomiphene citrate challenge test for ovarian reserve screening. Fertil Steril 1998;69:474–7.
37. Hendriks DJ, Mol BW, Bancsi LF, et al. The clomiphene citrate challenge test for the prediction of poor ovarian response and nonpregnancy in patients undergoing in vitro fertilization. a systematic review. Fertil Steril 2006;86: 807–18.
38. Hall JE, Welt CK, Cramer DW. Inhibin A and inhibin B reflect ovarian function in assisted reproduction but are less useful at predicting outcome. Hum Reprod 1999;14:409–15.

39. Muttukrishna S, McGarrigle H, Wakim R, et al. Antral follicle count, Antimullerian hormone and inhibin B: predictors of ovarian response in assisted reproductive technology? Br J Obstet Gynaecol 2005;112:1384–90.
40. de Vet A, Laven JS, de Jong FH, et al. Antimullerian hormone serum levels: a putative marker for ovarian aging. Fertil Steril 2002;77:357–62.
41. Wunder DM, Guibourdenche J, Birkhauser MH, et al. Anti-Mullerian hormone and inhibin B as predictors of pregnancy after treatment by in vitro fertilization/intra-cytoplasmic sperm injection. Fertil Steril 2008;90:2203–10.
42. Hehenkamp WJ, Looman CW, Themmen AP, et al. Anti-Mullerian hormone levels in the spontaneous menstrual cycle do not show substantial fluctuation. J Clin Endocrinol Metab 2006;91:4057–63.
43. Scheffer GJ, Broekmans FJ, Dorland M, et al. Antral follicle counts by transvaginal ultrasonography are related to age in women with proven natural fertility. Fertil Steril 1999;72:845–51.
44. Hendricks DJ, Mol BW, Bancsi LF, et al. Antral follicle count in the prediction of poor ovarian response and pregnancy after in vitro fertilization: a meta-analysis and comparison with basal follicle-stimulating hormone level. Fertil Steril 2005; 83:291–301.
45. Dolleman M, Faddy MJ, van Disseldorp J, et al. The relationship between anti-Mullerian hormone in women receiving fertility assessments and age at menopause in subfertile women: evidence from large population studies. J Clin Endocinol Metab 2013;98:1946–53.
46. Plante BJ, Beamon C, Schmitt CL, et al. Maternal antimullerian hormone levels do not predict fetal aneuploidy. J Assist Reprod Genet 2010;27:409–14.
47. Centers for Disease Control and Prevention, American Society for Reproductive Medicine Society for Assisted Reproductive Technology. 2011 assisted reproductive technology: National Summary Report. Atlanta (GA): Centers for Disease Control and Prevention; 2013.
48. Ziebe S, Loft A, Peterson JH, et al. Embryo quality and developmental potential is compromised by age. Acta Obstet Gynecol Scand 2001;80:169–74.
49. Hull MG, Fleming CF, Hughes AO, et al. The age related decline in female fecundity: a quantitative controlled study of implanting capacity and survival of individual embryos after in vitro fertilization. Fertil Steril 1996;65:783–90.
50. Scott RT, Ferry K, Su J, et al. Comprehensive chromosomal screening is highly predictive of the reproductive potential of human embryos: a prospective, blinded, nonselection study. Fertil Steril 2012;97:870–5.
51. Yeh JS, Steward RG, Dude AM, et al. Pregnancy outcomes decline in recipients over age 44: an analysis of 27,959 fresh donor oocyte in vitro fertilization cycles from the Society for Assisted Reproductive Technology. Fertil Steril 2014;101:1331–6.
52. Practice Committee of the American Society for Reproductive Medicine. Recommendations for gamete and embryo donation: a committee opinion. Fertil Steril 2013;99:47–62.
53. Practice Committee of the American Society for Reproductive Medicine. Repetitive oocyte donation. Fertil Steril 2006;86:S216–7.
54. Chang CC, Elliot TA, Wright G, et al. Prospective controlled study to evaluate laboratory and clinical outcomes of oocyte vitrification obtained in in vitro fertilization patients aged 30 to 39 years. Fertil Steril 2013;99:1891–7.
55. Lockwood GM. Social egg freezing: the prospect of reproductive 'immortality' or a dangerous delusion? Reprod Biomed Online 2011;23:334–40.
56. Cil AP, Bang K, Oktay K. Age specific probability of live birth with oocyte cryopreservation: an individual patient data meta-analysis. Fertil Steril 2013;100:492–9.

57. Odibo AO, Nelson D, Stamillo DM, et al. Advanced maternal age is an independent risk factor of intrauterine growth restriction. Am J Perinatol 2006;23:325–8.
58. Jacobsson B, Ladfors L, Milson I. Advanced maternal age and adverse perinatal outcome. Obstet Gynecol 2004;104:727–33.
59. Cleary-Goldman J, Malone FD, Vidaver J, et al. Impact of maternal age on obstetric outcome. Obstet Gynecol 2005;105:983–90.
60. Reddy UM, Ko C, Willinger M. Maternal age and the risk of stillbirth throughout pregnancy in the United States. Am J Obstet Gynecol 2006;195:764–70.
61. Naeye R. Maternal age, obstetric complications, and the outcome of pregnancy. Obstet Gynecol 1983;61:210–6.
62. Ethics Committee of the American Society for Reproductive Medicine. Oocyte or embryo donation to women of advanced age: a committee opinion. Fertil Steril 2013;100:337–40.

Ovulation Induction

Johanna Von Hofe, MD[a], G. Wright Bates, MD[b],*

KEYWORDS

- Ovulation induction • Clomiphene citrate • Letrozole • Gonadotropins
- Ovulation monitoring

KEY POINTS

- Before initiating ovulation induction, it is important to evaluate the underlying cause of a patient's anovulation and to make lifestyle modifications or treat underlying medical conditions, as appropriate.
- Clomiphene citrate has historically been the first-line treatment for patients with anovulatory infertility and can be used alone or with adjuvants.
- Recent evidence suggests that the aromatase inhibitor, letrozole, is the most effective oral agent for ovulation induction in women with polycystic ovarian syndrome.
- Exogenous gonadotropins may be required for women with hypothalamic hypogonadism and as an alternative to oral agents.
- Monitoring for an ovulatory response is imperative as it allows for appropriately timed intercourse or intrauterine insemination and assists in guiding alternative therapies when ovulation does not occur.

OVERVIEW

Ovulation induction is a phrase commonly used to describe the use of medication to stimulate normal ovulation in women with ovarian dysfunction. The medications used for ovulation induction can also promote follicular development or enhance ovulation in patients with other causes of infertility (male factor, age related, and unexplained), and they can be used to hyperstimulate ovaries for egg harvesting in assisted reproductive technologies or in vitro fertilization.[1]

Before initiating ovulation induction agents, it is important to evaluate the underlying cause of a patient's infertility with a complete history and physical examination. Laboratory evaluation and imaging with the following may be indicated:

- Thyroid-stimulating hormone with or without thyroid profile

The authors have nothing to disclose.
a Department of Obstetrics and Gynecology, University of Alabama Birmingham, Birmingham, AL 35249, USA; b Reproductive Endocrinology and Infertility, Department of Obstetrics and Gynecology, University of Alabama Birmingham, 1700 6th Avenue South, Room 10390, Birmingham, AL 35249, USA
* Corresponding author.
E-mail address: gbates@uabmc.edu

Obstet Gynecol Clin N Am 42 (2015) 27–37
http://dx.doi.org/10.1016/j.ogc.2014.09.007
0889-8545/15/$ – see front matter © 2015 Elsevier Inc. All rights reserved.

- Prolactin for pituitary disease
- Testosterone or androgen panel with clinical signs of androgen excess
- 17-hydroxy progesterone with suspicion for congenital adrenal hyperplasia
- Hemoglobin A1c with obesity or evidence of glucose intolerance
- Semen analysis
- Hysterosalpingogram, saline infusion sonogram or transvaginal ultrasound scan

After an initial evaluation, simple modifications such as weight loss (of 5%–10% of body weight in obese patients) or treatment of underlying endocrinopathies (in patients with thyroid disease, diabetes, hyperprolactinemia, or congenital adrenal hyperplasia) lead to the return of ovulation for some patients, thus, negating the need for ovulation induction agents.[2] For others, ovulation induction agents will be necessary, and a stepwise approach to treatment, coupled with appropriate monitoring and the strategic use of adjuvant therapies, lead to the practice of the most cost-effective, evidence-based medicine. Here, the agents commonly used for ovulation induction are reviewed with attention to their pharmacology, indications for use, therapy regimens, and efficacy.

CLOMIPHENE CITRATE
Pharmacology and Mechanism of Action

Clomiphene citrate (CC) is the oldest and most widely used ovulation induction agent. It is a nonsteroidal triphenylethylene derivative, which is structurally similar to estrogen, allowing it to bind competitively to the estrogen receptor (ER).[3] As a selective ER modulator (SERM), CC has both estrogen agonist and antagonist properties; however, it is the compound's agonist properties, which manifest in the setting of low endogenous estrogen levels, that are relevant in the setting of ovulation induction.[2]

When endogenous estrogen levels are low, CC competitively binds ERs throughout the reproductive system. CC also binds nuclear ERs for longer periods than endogenous estrogen, thus, depleting ER availability and falsely communicating a low estrogen state to the hypothalamus.[2] This, in turn, triggers natural compensatory mechanisms in the hypothalamic-pituitary-ovarian feedback axis, stimulating the body to alter pulsatile gonadotropin-releasing hormone (GnRH) secretion, which increases pituitary gonadotropin release and subsequently drives ovarian follicular activity.[3]

Indications for Use

The US Food and Drug Administration (FDA) approved CC for use in infertile patients with ovulatory dysfunction, and when combined with intrauterine insemination (IUI), CC has been found to be beneficial in patients with unexplained infertility. It is traditionally administered in a step-up regimen, and although it is highly efficacious in the appropriately selected patients, CC has significantly reduced efficacy when severe male factor, uterine, or tubal factors are also present.

Anovulatory infertility

CC has traditionally been the first-line treatment for anovulatory and oligo-ovulatory women.[3] Within this group, however, patients with hypogonadotropic hypogonadism, classified as World Health Organization (WHO) group I, and hypergonadotropic hypogonadism (WHO group III) are unlikely to respond. Patients with eugonadotropic hypogonadism (WHO group II) including those with polycystic ovarian syndrome (PCOS) comprise the largest percentage of anovulatory women seeking fertility care and are the most likely to benefit from CC.

The American Society for Reproductive Medicine and European Society for Human Reproduction and Embryology held a consensus conference in 2007 to establish specific guidelines for ovulation induction in women with PCOS. Their recommendations for treatment approach include CC as first-line therapy followed by gonadotropins and in vitro fertilization.[4]

A recent National Institutes of Health Consensus Conference on PCOS made the following observations about treatment of PCOS:

- Lifestyle modification and weight reduction
  - Decrease androgen effects
  - Increase ovulation
  - Improve insulin sensitivity
- Metformin
  - Decreases androgen expression
  - Modestly improves fertility
- Clomiphene and aromatase inhibitors
  - Increase fertility
- Gonadotropin therapy
  - Improves ovarian function (fertility)
  - Increases risks for multiple births and ovarian hyperstimulation syndrome[5]

Unexplained infertility

Clomiphene citrate is used empirically for the treatment of unexplained infertility, but there is currently no definitive evidence that it offers significant benefit over placebo alone in these patients.[6] However, when CC is used in combination with IUI, CC has shown a therapeutic benefit over placebo.[7]

Treatment Regimen and Efficacy

CC is administered orally beginning 2 to 5 days after the onset of a spontaneous or progestin-induced menses or arbitrarily in patients with amenorrhea with a negative pregnancy test result. Ovulation and pregnancy rates are similar regardless of whether CC is initiated on cycle day 2, 3, 4, or 5.[8]

Treatment typically begins with CC 50 mg daily for 5 days, and, if ovulation occurs, it is expected 5 to 10 days after the last dose of CC. It is important to monitor for ovulation in patients that are using CC to guide dosing adjustments, as CC should be continued at the lowest dose that achieves ovulation.

If the patient remains anovulatory at 50 mg/d, CC dosing may be titrated in 50-mg/d increments with each cycle until ovulation is achieved with standard effective doses ranging from 50 to 250 mg/d.

Fifty-two percent of women will ovulate in response to 50 mg of CC, and an additional 22% will respond to 100 mg.[9] There are varying opinions about maximum CC dosing, and although doses greater than 100 mg/d are not approved by the FDA, the American College of Obstetricians and Gynecologists supports doses of up to 150 mg/d before considering alternatives and recognizes that some women, particularly those with higher body mass indexes, will require higher doses to achieve ovulation.[10] One study has shown that CC-resistant women who fail to ovulate with a 5-day regimen of 250 mg/d may actually respond to an 8-day course of the same dose.[11] Doses up to 1000 mg and longer therapy duration have been described.

Among patients who do respond to CC, cycle fecundity approaches 15%, and cumulative pregnancy rates are as high as 75% over 6 to 9 cycles of treatment.[12,13] Similar to ovulatory women, the fecundity rate for women using CC decreases with age, and therapy for more than 6 cycles is not recommended, as increased duration of infertility is also associated with treatment failure.[2]

Tamoxifen, another SERM that is similar to CC in structure, has also proven successful as one ovulation induction agent with pregnancy rates as high as 40% in treatment-naïve patients and approaching 30% in CC-resistant patients.[14] The lack of superiority data and side effects, including hot flashes, limit its clinical utility.

ADJUVANT TREATMENT REGIMENS

Some women are resistant to CC but may ovulate with combined treatment regimens, specifically CC used in combination with glucocorticoids, exogenous human chorionic gonadotropin (hCG), or metformin.[2] Use of these adjuvants should be based on the patient's history, results of laboratory evaluation, and observations in previous unsuccessful CC treatment cycles. However, combination regimens should not be considered a prerequisite for use of more aggressive treatment strategies.[3]

Clomiphene and Glucocorticoids

In cases of CC resistance in the setting of normal and elevated dehydroepiandrosterone (DHEA) levels, the addition of daily dexamethasone (0.5–2 mg) or prednisone (5 mg) during the follicular phase (cycle days 5–14) to a CC regimen has shown an increase in ovulation and pregnancy rates when compared with CC plus placebo.[15–17] The largest randomized controlled trial studying this effect included 200 CC-resistant women and found a 10-fold increase in the cumulative pregnancy rate with the addition of dexamethasone (40%) compared with placebo (4%).[18]

The mechanism of the glucocorticoid effect has not been fully elucidated, but it is hypothesized that androgen suppression has direct effects on the oocyte and indirect effects on cytokines and intrafollicular growth factors.[19] Treatment is permissible for 3 to 6 cycles when ovulation is achieved but should be discontinued if not successful secondary to steroid side effects.

Clomiphene and Human Chorionic Gonadotropin

Patients using CC for ovulation induction for unexplained infertility or coexisting male factor infertility requiring IUI may benefit from an injection of hCG, used as a surrogate luteinizing hormone (LH) surge to trigger ovulation. However, a 2007 meta-analysis of 7 studies comparing trigger ovulation with urinary LH testing for IUI timing reported lower odds of pregnancy when an hCG trigger was used.[20] Therefore, exogenous hCG should be reserved for patients whose LH surge is not detected by ovulation predictor kits regardless of other objective evidence of ovulation.[2] In that select patient population, ultrasound evaluation is useful in determining when the hCG should be given (usually when the lead follicle diameter reaches 20–28 mm) so that IUI is appropriately timed (36 hours after hCG injection).[21,22]

Clomiphene and Metformin

The combination of metformin and CC deserves consideration in PCOS patients who are CC resistant before proceeding with alternative therapies. Data comparing CC and metformin as ovulation induction agents has been varied. The largest single trial comparing live birth rates in patients who took the 2 medications individually or in combination found that CC as a lone agent or in combination with metformin resulted in significantly higher birthrates (22.5% and 26.8%, respectively) than did metformin as a single agent (7.2%).[23] A few subsequent, small randomized controlled trials have found benefit in the addition of metformin to a CC regimen in PCOS patients who previously did not respond to CC alone in terms of ovulation and pregnancy rates.[3,24–26] If metformin is used, it is usually administered at 1500–2000 mg daily, which can be titrated up from a starting dose of 500 mg daily.

AROMATASE INHIBITORS
Pharmacology and Mechanism of Action

The aromatase inhibitors that are used for ovulation induction, anastrozole and letrozole, are triazole (antifungal) derivatives that function as competitive, nonsteroidal inhibitors of aromatase. When aromatase is blocked, androgens cannot be converted to estrogens, thereby creating a low estrogen state, releasing the hypothalamic-pituitary axis from the negative feedback of estrogen (**Fig. 1**). The body subsequently releases compensatory pulsatile GnRH, which increases pituitary gonadotropin release and subsequently drives ovarian follicular activity (as with CC).[2]

Although both CC and letrozole lead to increased GnRH secretion through negative feedback, their distinct mechanisms of action have functional and clinical importance.[27] Specifically, after letrozole treatment is ceased, estrogen levels increase immediately, which leads to a more abrupt decrease in follicle-stimulating hormone (FSH). This decrease makes gonadotropin support of multiples less likely, and the associated increase in estrogen allows for the production of cervical mucus and endometrial proliferation.

Indications for Use

Although aromatase inhibitors are FDA approved only in the treatment of postmenopausal breast cancer, they are increasingly used for ovulation induction based on their known mechanism of action (see previous discussion).[28]

Although CC has been used for several decades, letrozole may be the most effective oral agent for the treatment of anovulatory and unexplained infertility. Letrozole is clearly indicated in CC-resistant women or in those who are unable to use CC because of side effects, such as vasomotor symptoms, visual changes, or headaches.[29] Aromatase inhibitors should also be used in women who have a thin endometrium (<7 mm) when taking CC, as the proliferation of the endometrium is stimulated by estrogen, and letrozole does not have the same antiestrogen effects as CC.[30,31]

Therapy Regimen and Efficacy

Letrozole is typically administered at 2.7 to 7.5 mg daily, and the dose can be adjusted in 2.5-mg increments. Anastrozole is given as 1 mg daily. Both medications are administered in a very similar regimen to that of CC (for 5 days orally, usually starting on cycle day 3). Prolonged treatment courses (for 10 days) and single-dose regimens (20 mg once on cycle day 3), have been studied with some positive results.[32,33] However, most trials have focused on 2.5- and 5-mg doses of letrozole and 1-mg doses of anastrozole.

Letrozole can be used in conjunction with timed intercourse or IUI, and although it has been most studied in adjunct with hCG and ultrasonography, these additions are likely unnecessary in patients with ovulatory dysfunction who don't suffer from a secondary source of infertility (as with CC). Patients should be informed that letrozole is being prescribed off label so they can make an informed decision and are not concerned when they read the package instructions.

In anovulatory women who do not respond to CC treatment, aromatase inhibitors have been effective with a 60% ovulation rates and between a 12% and 40% pregnancy rates.[31,34]

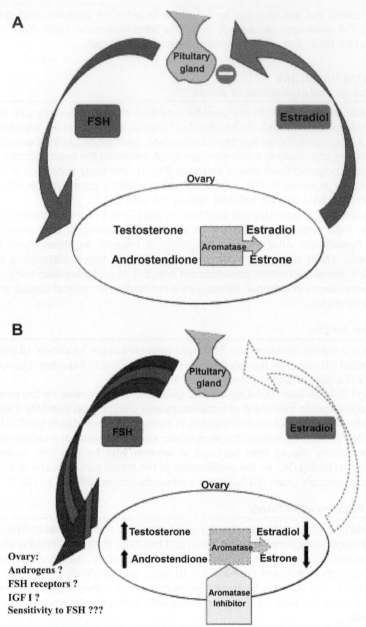

Fig. 1. Action of aromatase inhibitors. (*A*) The pituitary-ovarian axis in the follicular phase. Estradiol is produced by the ovarian granulosa cells and exerts a negative feedback effect on FSH release from the pituitary gland. (*B*) Effects of aromatase inhibitor. Aromatization of androgens to estrogens is inhibited, the hypothalamic-pituitary axis is released from the negative feedback, and FSH secretion is increased. The androgens accumulated in the ovary increase the ovarian sensitivity to FSH. The overall effect is stimulation of development of ovarian follicles. IGF I, insulin-like growth factor I. (*From* Holzer H, Casper R, Tulandi T. A new era in ovulation induction. Fertil Steril 2006;85:277; with permission.)

Three trials that used surrogate endpoints have compared aromatase inhibitors with CC in treatment-naïve anovulatory women in an effort to discern whether aromatase inhibitors might be considered a first-line treatment. The consensus based on those studies is that aromatase inhibitors may be as effective, but not more effective, than CC as ovulation induction agents.[35-37]

However, a recent, double-blind, multicenter trial, comparing letrozole with CC found that letrozole was associated with significantly higher cumulative live birth rates than CC (27.5% vs 19.1%, $P = .007$) without a higher incidence of congenital anomalies, pregnancy loss, or twin pregnancy. This landmark trial clearly suggests that letrozole is a better oral agent than clomiphene citrate for women with PCOS.[38]

EXOGENOUS GONADOTROPINS
Pharmacology and Mechanism of Action

Exogenous gonadotropins have evolved significantly over the last 25 years. Although the medications were historically prepared by purifying urine, many medications on the market today are the product of recombinant technology. Theoretic advantages of the new technology include more consistent supply, less variation in biologic activity, and the absence of antigenic urinary protein; however, based on available evidence, efficacy for ovulation induction may be similar regardless of preparation.[2,39] Because of their recombinant, bioactive subunits, exogenous gonadotropins function similarly to their natural counterparts.

Indications for Use

Hypogonadotropic hypogonadism
Oral ovulation induction agents are typically not effective in WHO group I patients, as those patients do not have intact hypothalamic-pituitary-ovarian axes. Exogenous gonadotropins restore normal cyclic ovulation for these patients and are considered first-line therapy.[40] Historically, GnRH was delivered in a pulsatile fashion via a pump, and although GnRH pump efficacy for monofollicular development was quite good, they had several limitations and are no longer available commercially.

Clomiphene citrate-resistant anovulation
As stated previously, exogenous gonadotropins are not considered first-line therapy for ovulation induction for most anovulatory patients and should only be considered in WHO II patients after a failure to respond to oral therapy.[4] PCOS is the most common diagnosis seen in this class, and these patients often display resistance to oral ovulation induction. However, gonadotropin therapy must be used with caution to avoid ovarian hyperstimulation syndrome and higher-order multiple pregnancies.

Unexplained infertility
Superovulation is often the goal of using gonadotropins in this population attempting to optimize cycle fecundity. This approach may be adopted after, or in lieu of, oral ovulation induction agents after appropriate patient education and counseling.

Therapy Regimen and Efficacy

Before initiating gonadotropins, the patient must understand the potential expense of medications and the commitment required to monitor medication effects. Close monitoring of serum estradiol levels and follicular number and growth by an experienced physician is mandatory to minimize risk.

The dose and duration of gonadotropin treatment required to induce ovulation varies and must be determined empirically. Each patient's response threshold is unpredictable, and although there is a relationship between body weight and dose requirement, body weight is not a reliable determinant of dosing.[41]

Hypogonadotropic hypogonadism

Urinary preparations, which contain both FSH and LH, are the medications of choice for these patients who (in theory) lack the necessary endogenous production of both gonadotropins. Many argue that these individuals also require luteal-phase support with hCG (2000–2500 IU every 3–4 days) or progesterone to compensate for low levels of endogenous LH. A step-up regimen should be used with initial doses of human menopausal gonadotropins (hMG) of as low as 75 IU daily. Doses are then adjusted based on the patient's monitored response and the goal of her therapy. When the dominant follicle measures 16 to 18 mm, hCG is given to trigger ovum release.[2]

Cycle fecundity in this patient population is greater than that observed in ovulating women at 25% with pregnancy rates after 6 cycles approaching 90%.[42]

Eugonadotropic hypogonadism

Because these patients often have normal levels of LH, there is a theoretic advantage of using only FSH to stimulate this group; however, multiple studies have found no difference in outcomes when comparing purified FSH preparations to hMG preparations. A step-up regimen should also be used for these patients with initial doses as low as 37.5 to 75 IU daily given these patients' tendencies to have several antral follicles and risk for ovarian hyperstimulation syndrome. Luteal support is seldom necessary.[43]

In CC-resistant women, cycle fecundity ranges from 5% to 15% with cumulative pregnancy rates in the 30% to 60 % range.[42]

Unexplained infertility

If superovulation is the goal—in an attempt to optimize cycle fecundity in older patients or those with unexplained infertility—higher daily doses of gonadotropins are

---

Box 1
Methods for monitoring ovulation

1. Basal body temperature recordings are an inexpensive method of detecting ovulation. However, because the temperature often increases only after the fertility window is closed and recordings can be tedious, this is not usually the preferred method of monitoring.[45]

2. Urine LH kits detect the endogenous LH surge that occurs 36 to 48 hours before ovulation.[46] This is an easy and reliable method and is generally the method of choice for patients who are on oral ovulation induction agents. After LH has been detected in the urine, patients should be instructed to have intercourse that day and the following day or schedule an IUI. In a cohort of women with no known obstacles to pregnancy, detection of ovulation and proper timing of intercourse doubled the chances of conception (odds ratio, 1.89).[47]

3. Luteal serum progesterone levels can also be measured to confirm that ovulation has occurred. A midluteal-phase serum progesterone should be greater than 3 ng/mL and preferably greater than 10 ng/mL. Serum progesterone should be measured approximately 1 week after expected ovulation. This will document ovulation but provides no guidance in the timing of intercourse or IUI.[48]

4. For patients that have difficulty detecting ovulation by ovulation predictor kits or who are using gonadotropins, ovarian follicular development can be monitored by ultrasound scan. This expensive and time consuming-endeavor should be avoided in patients for whom it is not necessary. When the lead follicle is 20 mm or more, ovulation can be induced with an injection of hCG. A recent retrospective study found higher pregnancy rates when the lead follicle was 23 to 28 mm when given hCG.[21] Intercourse or an IUI can be timed for 12 to 36 hours after the hCG injection.

usually given. This can be done with any of the available preparations and does not require luteal-phase support.[44]

Ovulation Induction Monitoring

When using medications for ovulation induction, monitoring for an ovulatory response is imperative, as it allows for appropriately timed intercourse or IUI and assists in guiding alternative therapies when ovulation does not occur. There are several methods to monitor ovulation, ranging from minimally invasive and inexpensive to invasive and expensive (**Box 1**).

REFERENCES

1. Cunningham FG, Williams JW. Williams obstetrics. 23rd edition. New York: McGraw-Hill Medical; 2010. xv, 1385.
2. Fritz MA, Speroff L. Clinical gynecologic endocrinology and infertility. 8th edition. Philadelphia: Wolters Kluwer Health/Lippincott Williams & Wilkins; 2011. x, 1439.
3. Practice Committee of the American Society for Reproductive Medicine. Use of clomiphene citrate in infertile women: a committee opinion. Fertil Steril 2013; 100(2):341–8.
4. Thessaloniki ESHRE/ASRM-Sponsored PCOS Consensus Workshop Group. Consensus on infertility treatment related to polycystic ovary syndrome. Fertil Steril 2008;89(3):505–22.
5. Amsterdam ESHRE/ASRM-Sponsored 3rd PCOS Consensus Workshop Group. Consensus on women's health aspects of polycystic ovary syndrome (PCOS). Hum Reprod 2012;27(1):14–24.
6. Guzick DS, Sullivan MW, Adamson GD, et al. Efficacy of treatment for unexplained infertility. Fertil Steril 1998;70(2):207–13.
7. Deaton JL, Gibson M, Blackmer KM, et al. A randomized, controlled trial of clomiphene citrate and intrauterine insemination in couples with unexplained infertility or surgically corrected endometriosis. Fertil Steril 1990;54(6):1083–8.
8. Wu CH, Winkel CA. The effect of therapy initiation day on clomiphene citrate therapy. Fertil Steril 1989;52(4):564–8.
9. Gorlitsky GA, Kase NG, Speroff L. Ovulation and pregnancy rates with clomiphene citrate. Obstet Gynecol 1978;51(3):265–9.
10. American College of Obstetricians and Gynecologists. ACOG practice bulletin. Management of infertility caused by ovulatory dysfunction. Number 34, February 2002. American College of Obstetricians and Gynecologists. Int J Gynaecol Obstet 2002;77(2):177–88.
11. Lobo RA, Granger LR, Davajan V, et al. An extended regimen of clomiphene citrate in women unresponsive to standard therapy. Fertil Steril 1982;37(6):762–6.
12. Imani B, Eijkemans MJ, te Velde ER, et al. Predictors of patients remaining anovulatory during clomiphene citrate induction of ovulation in normogonadotropic oligoamenorrheic infertility. J Clin Endocrinol Metab 1998;83(7):2361–5.
13. Imani B, Eijkemans MJ, te Velde ER, et al. Predictors of chances to conceive in ovulatory patients during clomiphene citrate induction of ovulation in normogonadotropic oligoamenorrheic infertility. J Clin Endocrinol Metab 1999;84(5): 1617–22.
14. Dhaliwal LK, Suri V, Gupta KR, et al. Tamoxifen: an alternative to clomiphene in women with polycystic ovary syndrome. J Hum Reprod Sci 2011;4(2):76–9.
15. Daly DC, Walters CA, Soto-Albors CE, et al. A randomized study of dexamethasone in ovulation induction with clomiphene citrate. Fertil Steril 1984;41(6):844–8.

16. Lobo RA, Paul W, March CM, et al. Clomiphene and dexamethasone in women unresponsive to clomiphene alone. Obstet Gynecol 1982;60(4):497–501.
17. Trott EA, Plouffe L Jr, Hansen K, et al. Ovulation induction in clomiphene-resistant anovulatory women with normal dehydroepiandrosterone sulfate levels: beneficial effects of the addition of dexamethasone during the follicular phase. Fertil Steril 1996;66(3):484–6.
18. Parsanezhad ME, Alborzi S, Motazedian S, et al. Use of dexamethasone and clomiphene citrate in the treatment of clomiphene citrate-resistant patients with polycystic ovary syndrome and normal dehydroepiandrosterone sulfate levels: a prospective, double-blind, placebo-controlled trial. Fertil Steril 2002;78(5):1001–4.
19. Keay SD, Jenkins JM. Adjunctive use of dexamethasome in Clomid resistant patients. Fertil Steril 2003;80(1):230–1 [author reply: 231].
20. Kosmas IP, Tatsioni A, Fatemi HM, et al. Human chorionic gonadotropin administration vs. luteinizing monitoring for intrauterine insemination timing, after administration of clomiphene citrate: a meta-analysis. Fertil Steril 2007;87(3):607–12.
21. Palatnik A, Strawn E, Szabo A, et al. What is the optimal follicular size before triggering ovulation in intrauterine insemination cycles with clomiphene citrate or letrozole? An analysis of 988 cycles. Fertil Steril 2012;97(5):1089–94.e1-3.
22. Andersen AG, Als-Nielsen B, Hornnes PJ, et al. Time interval from human chorionic gonadotrophin (HCG) injection to follicular rupture. Hum Reprod 1995;10(12):3202–5.
23. Legro RS, Barnhart HX, Schlaff WD, et al. Clomiphene, metformin, or both for infertility in the polycystic ovary syndrome. N Engl J Med 2007;356(6):551–66.
24. Hwu YM, Lin SY, Huang WY, et al. Ultra-short metformin pretreatment for clomiphene citrate-resistant polycystic ovary syndrome. Int J Gynaecol Obstet 2005;90(1):39–43.
25. Sahin Y, Yirmibes U, Kelestimur F, et al. The effects of metformin on insulin resistance, clomiphene-induced ovulation and pregnancy rates in women with polycystic ovary syndrome. Eur J Obstet Gynecol Reprod Biol 2004;113(2):214–20.
26. Vandermolen DT, Ratts VS, Evans WS, et al. Metformin increases the ovulatory rate and pregnancy rate from clomiphene citrate in patients with polycystic ovary syndrome who are resistant to clomiphene citrate alone. Fertil Steril 2001;75(2):310–5.
27. Holzer H, Casper R, Tulandi T. A new era in ovulation induction. Fertil Steril 2006; 85(2):277–84.
28. Speroff L, Fritz MA. Clinical gynecologic endocrinology and infertility. 7th edition. Philadelphia: Lippincott Williams & Wilkins; 2005. x, 1334.
29. Nahid L, Sirous K. Comparison of the effects of letrozole and clomiphene citrate for ovulation induction in infertile women with polycystic ovary syndrome. Minerva Ginecol 2012;64(3):253–8.
30. Mitwally MF, Casper RF. Use of an aromatase inhibitor for induction of ovulation in patients with an inadequate response to clomiphene citrate. Fertil Steril 2001; 75(2):305–9.
31. Begum MR, Ferdous J, Begum A, et al. Comparison of efficacy of aromatase inhibitor and clomiphene citrate in induction of ovulation in polycystic ovarian syndrome. Fertil Steril 2009;92(3):853–7.
32. Badawy A, Mosbah A, Tharwat A, et al. Extended letrozole therapy for ovulation induction in clomiphene-resistant women with polycystic ovary syndrome: a novel protocol. Fertil Steril 2009;92(1):236–9.
33. Mitwally MF, Casper RF. Single-dose administration of an aromatase inhibitor for ovarian stimulation. Fertil Steril 2005;83(1):229–31.
34. Atay V, Cam C, Muhcu M, et al. Comparison of letrozole and clomiphene citrate in women with polycystic ovaries undergoing ovarian stimulation. J Int Med Res 2006;34(1):73–6.

35. Bayar U, Basaran M, Kiran S, et al. Use of an aromatase inhibitor in patients with polycystic ovary syndrome: a prospective randomized trial. Fertil Steril 2006; 86(5):1447–51.
36. Badawy A, Abdel Aal I, Abulatta M. Clomiphene citrate or letrozole for ovulation induction in women with polycystic ovarian syndrome: a prospective randomized trial. Fertil Steril 2009;92(3):849–52.
37. Badawy A, Abdel Aal I, Abulatta M. Clomiphene citrate or anastrozole for ovulation induction in women with polycystic ovary syndrome? A prospective controlled trial. Fertil Steril 2009;92(3):860–3.
38. Legro RS, Brzyski RG, Diamond MP, et al. Letrozole versus clomiphene for infertility in the polycystic ovary syndrome. N Engl J Med 2014;371(2):119–29.
39. Lathi RB, Milki AA. Recombinant gonadotropins. Curr Womens Health Rep 2001; 1(2):157–63.
40. Agents stimulating gonadal function in the human. Report of a WHO scientific group. World Health Organ Tech Rep Ser 1973;514:1–30.
41. Chong AP, Rafael RW, Forte CC. Influence of weight in the induction of ovulation with human menopausal gonadotropin and human chorionic gonadotropin. Fertil Steril 1986;46(4):599–603.
42. Balen AH, Braat DDM, West C, et al. Cumulative conception and live birth rates after the treatment of anovulatory infertility: safety and efficacy of ovulation induction in 200 patients. Hum Reprod 1994;9(8):1563–70.
43. Nugent D, Vanderkerchove P, Hughes E, et al. Gonadotrophin therapy for ovulation induction in subfertility associated with polycystic ovary syndrome. Cochrane Database Syst Rev 2000;(4):CD000410.
44. Dodson WC, Haney AF. Controlled ovarian hyperstimulation and intrauterine insemination for treatment of infertility. Fertil Steril 1991;55(3):457–67.
45. Practice Committee of the American Society for Reproductive Medicine. Use of clomiphene citrate in women. Fertil Steril 2006;86(5 Suppl 1):S187–93.
46. Practice Committee of American Society for Reproductive Medicine in collaboration with Society for Reproductive Endocrinology and Infertility. Optimizing natural fertility. Fertil Steril 2008;90(Suppl 5):S1–6.
47. Robinson J, Wakelin M, Ellis J. Increased pregnancy rate with use of the Clearblue Easy Fertility Monitor. Fertil Steril 2007;2:329–34.
48. Wathen NC, Perry L, Lilford RJ, et al. Interpretation of single progesterone measurement in diagnosis of anovulation and defective luteal phase: observations on analysis of the normal range. Br Med J (Clin Res Ed) 1984;288(6410):7–9.

Fertility Preservation in the Age of Assisted Reproductive Technologies

Paul R. Brezina, MD, MBA[a,b,c],*, William H. Kutteh, MD, PhD[a,b,c],
Amelia P. Bailey, MD[c], Jianchi Ding, PhD[d],
Raymond W. Ke, MD[a,b,c], James L. Klosky, PhD[e]

KEYWORDS

- Fertility preservation • Cryopreservation • Freezing • Egg • Sperm • Oocyte
- Cancer • Oncology

KEY POINTS

- Strategies used to accomplish fertility preservation are many.
- Over the past several decades, new technologies, especially related to assisted reproductive technologies and in vitro fertilization, have greatly expanded ways to accomplish fertility preservation. These advances have also grown the indications for pursing fertility potential in general.
- Surely, advances in technology will continue to be optimized in the future.
- By all indicators, the role for fertility preservation in society and medicine is likely to only increase over the next several decades.

The authors have no pertinent disclosures and conflicts of interest.
Sources of Funding: None.
Contributors: P.R. Brezina, A.P. Bailey, R.W. Ke, J.L. Klosky, and W.H. Kutteh primarily searched the literature and wrote the first draft of the article; P.R. Brezina is guarantor.
Competing Interests: All authors have completed the Unified Competing Interest form and declare no support from any organization for the submitted work, no financial relationships with any organizations that might have an interest in the submitted work in the previous 3 years, and no other relationships or activities that could appear to have influenced the submitted work.

[a] Vanderbilt University School of Medicine, 1161 21st Avenue South, R-1200 Medical Center North, Nashville, TN 37232-2521, USA; [b] Department of Surgery, St. Jude Children's Research Hospital, 262 Danny Thomas Place, Memphis, TN 38105-3678, USA; [c] Fertility Associates of Memphis, 80 Humphreys Center, Suite 307, Memphis, TN 38120-2363, USA; [d] IVF Laboratory, Fertility Associates of Memphis, 80 Humphreys Center, Suite 307, Memphis, TN 38120, USA; [e] Cancer Survivorship, St. Jude Children's Research Hospital, 262 Danny Thomas Place–MS 740, Memphis, TN 38105-3678, USA
* Corresponding author. Vanderbilt University School of Medicine, 1161 21st Avenue South, R-1200 Medical Center North, Nashville, TN 37232-2521.
E-mail address: pbrezina@fertilitymemphis.com

Obstet Gynecol Clin N Am 42 (2015) 39–54
http://dx.doi.org/10.1016/j.ogc.2014.09.004
0889-8545/15/$ – see front matter © 2015 Elsevier Inc. All rights reserved.

INTRODUCTION

Reproduction has been and will always be central to the human experience. Many individuals experience situations that may compromise their future fertility. The reasons for this are many, ranging from social pressure to defer childbearing, to exposure to gonadotoxic agents (eg, chemotherapy) that damage reproductive organs. Both men and women may be placed in environments that could compromise their future fertility.

Historically, the options for preserving fertility were quite limited. Women could choose to have children earlier in life than they would have ideally chosen at the possible expense of their careers. Men known to have a malignancy could undergo cryopreservation (freezing) of their sperm before being exposed to caustic chemotherapy. Barring these 2 approaches, the options for fertility preservation, particularly for women, have been quite limited.

The past several decades, however, have seen technologies that have changed the historical limitations regarding fertility preservation. Assisted reproductive technologies (ART) associated specifically with in vitro fertilization (IVF) have ushered in new tools that are now routinely used to preserve fertility. Cryopreservation of unfertilized eggs and embryos gives a new set of options for women desiring fertility preservation for a variety of indications. An outline of available technologies currently used for fertility preservation is shown in **Box 1**. In addition, the use of surgical, medical, pharmacologic, and psychological interventions offer mechanisms to facilitate fertility preservation, particularly in the setting of oncology. This review attempts to offer an overview of the state of the art within fertility preservation.

CRYOPRESERVATION TECHNOLOGIES AVAILABLE
Sperm Cryopreservation

The ability to cryopreserve human sperm was first established in 1953 in a report by Bunge and Sherman.[1] Since this time, the use of sperm cryopreservation has become the dominant method of fertility preservation for men faced with fertility challenges.[2]

The process of performing sperm cryopreservation is relatively straightforward. Sperm is classically obtained through masturbation.[3] In some cases in which sperm is not possible to be obtained through ejaculation, surgical techniques also exist that may retrieve sperm for cryopreservation.[3] The semen obtained is then allowed to liquefy at room temperature and analyzed for motility, concentration, and morphology.[3] Following this, many centers will use a selection process such as a swim-up or density gradient centrifugation to identify the most viable sperm within the sample, which is then cryopreserved.[3] Cryopreserved sperm are considered relatively stable and may be used even decades later to result in pregnancy.[4]

Some studies have noted DNA damage to some but not all sperm following cryopreservation.[5] However, the safety of using cryopreserved sperm to achieve pregnancy is generally accepted, as decades of healthy pregnancies have resulted from cryopreserved sperm.[3,6] Once thawed, sperm may be used to achieve pregnancy either through intrauterine insemination techniques or through IVF.

A common indication for sperm cryopreservation is fertility preservation in the setting of cancer. Current recommendations from multiple professional societies recommend that men diagnosed with cancer should universally be offered sperm cryopreservation before initiation of treatment with chemotherapy or radiation that could reasonably impact sperm production.[6,7] However, using sperm cryopreservation in

Box 1
Available fertility preservation strategies

- Cryopreservation Technologies
  - Sperm Cryopreservation
    - Advantages
      - Easy to obtain in most patients
      - Excellent results
      - Long track record
    - Disadvantages
      - Only possible in male patients
  - Embryo Cryopreservation
    - Advantages
      - Excellent results in young patients
      - Long track record
    - Disadvantages
      - Requires in vitro fertilization (IVF) to obtain eggs
      - May be financially costly
      - Requires female patients to choose sperm donor before cryopreservation
  - Oocyte Cryopreservation
    - Advantages
      - Excellent results in young patients
      - Does not require female patients to choose sperm donor before cryopreservation
    - Disadvantages
      - Requires IVF to obtain eggs
      - May be financially costly
      - Relatively short track record
- Surgical Technologies
  - Ovarian Transposition
    - Advantages
      - Proven benefit in certain clinical situations
      - Does not require female patients to choose sperm donor before cryopreservation
    - Disadvantages
      - Requires surgery
      - May not have return to baseline fertility potential after radiation
  - Uterine Transplantation
    - Advantages
      - Preserves hope of carrying a child for some women in whom uterine function is not adequate to achieve a healthy pregnancy
    - Disadvantages
      - Requires surgery
      - Considered experimental at the present time

- Medical Technologies
  - Use of gonadotropin-releasing hormone agonists
    - Advantages
      - Not difficult to perform
      - Relatively inexpensive
      - Does not require female patients to choose sperm donor before cryopreservation
    - Disadvantages
      - May not have return to baseline fertility potential after radiation

the setting of cancer therapy is currently underused, with many patients never being offered fertility preservation before oncologic treatment.[3] Chemotherapy and radiation treatments have unpredictable impacts on subsequent sperm production.[3,7] However, the potential for such treatments conferring a deleterious effect on sperm production and quality is not questioned.[3,7] The posthumous use of sperm after fertility preservation also has been described and informed written consent regarding this topic should be obtained at the time of sperm collection for cryopreservation.[8]

The use of sperm cryopreservation is not exclusive to the setting of cancer. Men with a suboptimal semen analysis may elect to cryopreserve a sperm sample before proceeding with fertility treatments as an "insurance policy" should semen parameters continue to decline in the future. Additionally, the use of donor sperm obtained from large sperm cryobanks is common in the fertility treatment of women wishing to achieve pregnancy in the setting of male factor infertility or when there is no male partner.[9]

OOCYTE AND EMBRYO CRYOPRESERVATION
Available Technology

The first successful report of an IVF procedure was published in *The Lancet* by Drs Steptoe and Edwards in 1978.[10] This procedure is performed by surgically removing periovulatory oocytes from a woman, fertilizing the obtained eggs, and growing resulting embryos in a laboratory environment. Embryo(s) may be then placed in the uterus, resulting in the possibility of pregnancy.

Within a decade, techniques designed to achieve multifollicular development of ovarian oocytes in an IVF cycle, a process known as controlled ovarian hyperstimulation (COH), were well described.[11] COH allowed women to obtain many eggs during a single IVF egg retrieval.[11] This led to experimentation with cryopreserving embryos for use at a later time. By the mid-1980s, pregnancies resulting from the transfer of cryopreserved embryos, a procedure known as frozen embryo transfer, were being reported.[12]

The process of freezing embryos has become increasingly sophisticated with time. One of the chief dangers involved in embryo cryopreservation is the formation of ice crystals during the freezing process that may cause irreparable damage to cellular structures.[13] Consequently, techniques that have been developed for embryo cryopreservation attempt to minimize this phenomenon. Cryoprotective additives are used to dehydrate embryonic cells before cryopreservation, thus reducing intracellular ice crystal formation.[12,13] Traditionally, embryos were cryopreserved using a process called slow cooling. Slow cooling uses a low cooling rate of approximately 0.3°C per minute until the temperature of approximately −40°C is achieved, at which point the rate of cooling is accelerated to approximately 50°C per minute to a goal storing temperature of −100° to −150°C.[12–14]

Although many centers described success in the slow cooling of embryos, a more recent technique introduced in the early 2000s, known as vitrification, is now widely accepted by many experts as the gold standard for embryo cryopreservation.[15] Vitrification uses extremely rapid cooling rates of more than 10,000°C per minute and uses specialized carrier systems (open vs closed).[12,15,16] Vitrification accomplishes a near "glasslike" crystal lattice within the cryopreserved embryo, which is thought to dramatically decrease the chances for ice crystal formation.[13,17] Embryo survival and pregnancy rates from embryos, particularly at the blastocyst stage, may be superior using vitrification as compared with slow freezing.[16] Consequently, a general shift toward increased use of vitrification has occurred in many centers.[18] However, some data show that in the right hands, similar outcomes exist with vitrification and slow freezing.[19,20] Therefore, the superiority of a single cryopreserving modality remains somewhat controversial.

Successful oocyte cryopreservation using slow freezing techniques has been described for several decades.[21] However, the rate of survival on thawing oocytes frozen using slow freezing techniques and correlating pregnancy rates were disappointing.[13,21] These suboptimal results using slow freezing resulted in classifying oocyte cryopreservation as experimental. Recently, vitrification technology has been applied to oocyte cryopreservation. Pregnancy rates using oocyte cryopreservation using vitrification have been extremely encouraging, and protocols for optimizing this practice are now well described.[22] In 2013, the American Society of Reproductive Medicine removed the "experimental" label associated with oocyte cryopreservation.[23] After this, the American College of Obstetricians and Gynecologists confirmed that oocyte cryopreservation was no longer considered experimental.[24] Oocyte cryopreservation is now considered a mainstream technology that is commonly used under the umbrella of ART and IVF.[25]

ONCOLOGIC APPLICATIONS

Annually in the United States, more than 130,000 patients are diagnosed with cancer in their reproductive years (up to 45 years), including more than 12,000 children (0–19 years).[26] With modern, comprehensive treatment, the vast majority of children, adolescents, and young adults diagnosed with cancer will become long-term survivors.[26,27] Combined with a trend in delayed childbearing, fertility after cancer treatment has become a key quality-of-life issue to many patients (and their parents) in this age group. Unfortunately, fertility in both male and female survivors appears to be compromised, particularly if alkylating agents and/or radiation were administered.[28] Among young patients with cancer, the ability to preserve fertility options before gonadotoxic treatment has become of paramount importance.[7] For pubertal girls, retrieving oocytes for both oocyte or embryo cryopreservation is valid and should be offered, but it is also time-consuming and necessitates a quick decision when the patient may already be overwhelmed by a multitude of other management issues, including impending cancer treatments. Finally, access to fertility preservation services because of availability and cost is still variable across the United States.[7]

Fertility preservation via either oocyte or embryo cryopreservation is an increasingly used strategy in the setting of oncology.[25] The ovaries have long been known to be exquisitely sensitive to damage from exposure to cancer treatments such as chemotherapy or radiation therapy.[29] Damage from these agents has been well documented for decades to lead to damage that in many cases results in amenorrhea and the complete failure of competent follicular recruitment and ovulation.[29]

However, the fecundity rates after significant ovarian exposure to these agents may be significantly lower than background even when menses continue or return.[30] Many experts now believe that damage to core mechanisms within the oocytes themselves, possibly on a genetic level, is the cause of these long-term compromised fecundity rates. Some chemotherapy agents, such as alkylating drugs, are known to confer a greater deleterious effect than other agents, such as methotrexate.[31] However, the true extent of damage from all chemotherapy agents has not yet been fully described. Similarly, cancer therapies using radiation can exert a deleterious effect, but the extent of this damage is not fully defined.

Embryo and oocyte cryopreservation represent an accessible technology with which women may pursue fertility preservation before oncologic treatments. Cryopreserved oocytes or embryos may be used once a cancer-free status is achieved if there is no residual ovarian function after therapy. Sadly, however, cryopreservation strategies in the setting of cancer therapy are currently underused, with many patients not receiving adequate counseling on fertility preservation before oncologic treatment.[16,31,32] Recently, opinions from major professional societies state that the current standard of care should include offering fertility preservation to patients faced with oncologic treatment.[7,16,31,32]

At St Jude Children's Research Hospital, an increased focus for offering fertility preservation is taking place among adolescent and young adult patients at increased risk for infertility secondary to cancer treatment. Before, during, and even after receiving chemotherapy and radiation treatments for hematologic/oncologic diseases, St Jude patients are now routinely offered a consultation with a board-certified reproductive endocrinologist from our center. After considering available options, many patients then choose to proceed with fertility preservation through either sperm cryopreservation or through ovulation induction with oocyte cryopreservation. This practice has given hope of retained fertility to many young men and women, and we are optimistic that this sort of progressive program will be adopted by other centers on a large scale.

WOMEN WISHING TO PRESERVE THEIR FERTILITY POTENTIAL

For thousands of years, there was essentially no mechanism other than abstinence with which human beings could control the timing of reproduction. This resulted in women undergoing childbearing relatively early in their lives. Today, many perceive this early childbearing to functionally conflict with career advancement for many women. The introduction of oral birth control pills as a form of contraception in the 1960s fundamentally altered this paradigm and afforded women the power to control their fertility and delay childbearing. As a result, the age at which women achieve pregnancy has continually and significantly increased since the 1960s, especially in wealthy nations.[33]

Unfortunately, fertility potential in women decreases with age, especially after the age of 35. Many women who would be mildly subfertile in their 20s are unable to achieve pregnancy via natural intercourse alone in their mid-late 30s and early 40s.[23,34,35] Consequently, the use of ARTs, such as IVF, to achieve pregnancy is relatively common in this age group. However, even with such measures, pregnancy rates per month are low, generally not exceeding 10% per IVF attempt, after the age of 42. Therefore, for many women, delaying childbearing until their late 30s or early 40s results in a significantly lower possibility for achieving pregnancy with their biological child.

The first pregnancies resulting from cryopreserved oocytes and embryos were reported in the mid-1980s.[23,36] Although pregnancy rates associated with embryo cryopreservation were encouraging, survival rates of cryopreserved oocytes were generally poor.[37] Therefore, for the past several decades, a solution to minimize the effect of maternal age on fertility decline has been to undergo an IVF cycle, cryopreserve embryos, and place these embryos into the uterus at the time pregnancy is desired. Because fertility for the most part is felt to be tied to ovarian age, rather than the age of the uterus, pregnancy rates using this approach were encouraging.

A central limitation of embryo cryopreservation, however, is that this approach requires women to choose a male sperm donor to fertilize an oocyte (egg) before cryopreservation. Early attempts to freeze unfertilized oocytes were generally discouraging and not felt to be optimal for fertility preservation by many experts.[37] Although embryo cryopreservation did offer a viable option for fertility preservation in some couples, this option was unappealing for some women who did not have a male partner at the time of desired fertility preservation.[19] Following the description of excellent pregnancy rates using vitrification techniques to cryopreserve oocytes, dozens of centers began to use this technology on a routine basis. Currently, pregnancy success rates from IVF cycles using oocyte cryopreservation are comparable to fresh IVF cycles, a feat that has been realized only in the past several years.[13,22]

The ability to efficiently and effectively cryopreserve oocytes has the potential to have a significant social impact over the next several decades. Before this technology, women entering their mid to late 30s electing to defer pregnancy accepted a continually declining age-related fertility potential and the possibility of not ever having their own genetic child. Oocyte cryopreservation empowers women to delay childbearing without committing, at the time of the procedure, to what sperm will be ultimately used for fertilization. Some have compared the ultimate social impact of oocyte cryopreservation to the introduction of birth control pills.[25] Oocyte cryopreservation also has other applications. This technology is likely to emerge as a central tool for preserving fertility in young oncology patients who have not initiated or completed childbearing. Additionally, couples undergoing IVF who have ethical or moral objections to cryopreserving embryos may avoid this concern with oocyte freezing.

Leading centers around the world now routinely offer oocyte cryopreservation for fertility preservation. Over the past several years, oocyte cryopreservation has become increasingly visible in the public eye. Multiple high-profile celebrities have publically announced that they are pursing or have undergone oocyte cryopreservation for fertility preservation.[25] This procedure is appropriate for young women wishing to maximize their future fertility when achieving pregnancy is not desired until the mid to late 30s or beyond.

Because the sharpest decline in a woman's fertility occurs after the age of 35, oocyte cryopreservation is most effective if pursued at a relatively young age, ideally before the age of 30.[23,24] In healthy women, it is believed that the average chance of achieving a pregnancy from one mature egg is approximately 5% to 10%.[19,38] Therefore, on average, freezing 10 to 12 mature eggs from a young woman generally provides a good statistical chance for achieving pregnancy up to the late 40s. Ultimate pregnancy rates resulting from oocyte cryopreservation are known to most sharply decline after the age of 38.[39] Although obtaining this number of eggs is common in young women, some women may require multiple IVF stimulation cycles to "bank" this number of oocytes. Therefore, oocyte cryopreservation cannot ensure future fertility. Rather, this strategy serves as an "insurance policy" that could be used if pregnancy with natural intercourse is not achieved at the desired time in the future. Women interested in oocyte cryopreservation are encouraged to discuss the capabilities and limitations of the procedure with a physician specializing in ARTs.

COUPLES UNDERGOING IN VITRO FERTILIZATION WITH ETHICAL OR MORAL CONCERNS

Some couples undergoing IVF are concerned about freezing additional embryos that may not be used in the future.[24] As an alternative, in the course of an IVF cycle, it is now possible to fertilize fewer oocytes, which could become embryos, while cryopreserving the excess unfertilized oocytes. This approach allows couples to sequentially thaw and fertilize oocytes to generate the number of embryos necessary to achieve their reproductive goals. Excess unfertilized oocytes may then be donated or discarded when the couple's family is complete.

WOMEN WITH CERTAIN GENETIC CONDITIONS

Several genetic disorders have been associated with early ovarian failure. For example, women with fragile X premutation or mosaic Turner syndrome may choose to cryopreserve oocytes while they still have ovarian function. Other genetic mutations, such as the BRCA mutations, are associated with an increased risk of ovarian cancer. Women who elect to have prophylactic salpingo-oophorectomy may choose to cryopreserve oocytes before surgery.

OVARIAN TRANSPOSITION

The effects of radiation on fertility are dependent on patient age, dosage, interval between doses, disease type and location, and size of the radiation field. Standard radiation doses are 40 to 50 Gy; however, higher doses are given in total-body irradiation protocols before bone marrow transplantation, as would be required for treatment of recurrent lymphoma or leukemia.[40,41] Ovarian failure is seen in more than 90% of patients receiving at least 5 Gy of pelvic radiation.[42] Further, scatter radiation from a beam not aimed directly at the pelvis may still impact future reproduction.[43] Less extensive radiation fields and minimal doses carry a lower risk of infertility,[44] and several studies show that doses less than 5 Gy do not decrease fertility.[45–47] However, due to lower ovarian reserve, increasing age at the time of radiation is related to greater gonadotoxicity, just as with chemotherapy.

Oophoropexy and ovarian transposition are procedures that change the location of the ovaries in an attempt to remove them from the pelvic radiation field. They differ only in their surgical technique, so herein the terms will be used interchangeably. These procedures may be used to lessen the likelihood of scatter radiation affecting the ovaries in gynecologic as well as colorectal and spinal cancers for which radiation is planned.[48] Ovarian transposition may be performed either at the time of laparotomy if one is needed for treatment or may be done laparoscopically in the outpatient setting as an isolated procedure. Oophoropexy can reduce ovarian radiation dose up to 95%.[49] Because the ovaries remain on their original attachments, they can migrate back to the pelvis. So, oophoropexy should be conducted immediately before radiation treatment begins.[50] If chemotherapy that is not gonadotoxic is planned before pelvic irradiation, the procedure should be performed before initiation of chemotherapy. This is because patients are immunosuppressed on most chemotherapeutic regimens and, therefore, may not be healthy enough to undergo elective surgery.

Ovarian transposition is not indicated if gonadotoxic chemotherapy is planned, because the ovaries will be adversely affected by the medication regardless of their location.

After transposition, 60% to 89% of patients with cancer who are younger than 40 maintain ovarian function.[50–53] Failures are a result of radiation that scatters to the new ovarian location as well as necrosis of the ovary from compromised blood supply due to transposition, as necrosis can lead to follicular atresia and premature menopause.[54–58] Most women retain enough ovarian tissue for endocrine function, but some studies report that only 15% of patients are fertile after ovarian transposition.[59]

Spontaneous pregnancies have been reported after oophoropexy. However, some patients need either oocyte retrieval with in vitro fertilization or reversal of the procedure because the ovary is no longer in close proximity to the fallopian tube.[56,60] Transvaginal oocyte retrieval is more difficult after transposition due to increased distance between the vagina and ovary.[56] Transabdominal aspiration may be attempted, but that approach can yield fewer oocytes.[49] However, one publication revealed no significant differences between transvaginal and transabdominal aspiration in the number of damaged oocytes, fertilization rates, embryo number and quality, and clinical and ongoing pregnancy rates.[61]

Additional complications may arise after oophoropexy, such as pelvic pain from ovarian or fallopian tube infarction or cyst formation. Further, ovarian cancer detection by physical examination is more difficult if the ovaries are no longer located in the pelvis.[62] Gonadal shielding can reduce the radiation dose to the ovaries if ovarian transposition is contraindicated for any reason, but this technique is possible only with certain radiation fields and requires significant expertise in this area.[62]

UTERINE TRANSPLANTATION

After a hysterectomy for gynecologic cancer, uterine transplantation as part of a research study is the only way a patient could carry a pregnancy. The first transplantation of a human uterus resulting in patient survival was performed in Saudi Arabia in 2000. Unfortunately, the uterus had to be removed 99 days after surgery due to necrosis from clotting in the uterine vessels.[63] Despite this failure, great strides have been made in the area due to advances in antirejection regimens, and the first successful transplantation was performed in 2011 in Turkey.[64] The patient conceived in 2013, but the pregnancy failed in the first trimester.[65] Also in 2013, 9 Swedish women received uterine transplants and had subsequent menstrual cycles, but there are no reported pregnancies yet.[66] Posttransplantation pregnancies have been demonstrated in mice and dogs with birth by cesarean delivery in sheep.[67–71] Uterine transplantation is considered investigational in humans at this time, but advances in the field have been significant over the past 2 decades.

USE OF GONADOTROPIN-RELEASING HORMONE AGONISTS IN THE SETTING OF ONCOFERTILITY

Radiation and chemotherapeutic agents act on rapidly dividing cells, such as those encountered in malignancies and gonadal germ cells. In female individuals, ovarian primordial follicles and oocytes are particularly sensitive to cytotoxic agents. These germ cell complexes cannot be replenished, and their destruction may lead to premature ovarian failure, a condition commonly referred to as premature menopause. Although age-dependent, up to two-thirds of all women treated for cancer will develop premature menopause.[72] Administration of gonadotropin-releasing hormone analogs

(GnRHa) to suppress pituitary gonadotropins and follicle-stimulating hormone (FSH)-dependent germ cell maturation theoretically would prevent ovarian follicle maturation and destruction. However, the initial differentiation of primordial follicles is not FSH-dependent, thus potentially limiting the protective effect of GnRHa in female individuals. In mouse models, prepubertal status has not been protective against the follicle depletion induced by cyclophosphamide at doses similar to those used therapeutically in humans.[73]

In female individuals, most prospective studies investigating gonadal protection by GnRHa during chemotherapy were uncontrolled and demonstrated inconsistent results. Almost all have used resumption of menses as the primary outcome. Unfortunately, return of menstruation and ovulation is a poor marker of fertility, as successful gestation requires the release of a robust, high-quality oocyte. It is likely that these high-quality oocytes would be the most susceptible to chemotherapy-induced cytotoxicity.[73]

Despite these concerns, there is level I evidence supporting the use of GnRHa suppression before chemotherapy to preserve ovarian function. An Italian study randomized 282 premenopausal women with breast cancer to receive chemotherapy with or without triptorelin, a depot GnRHa. One year after chemotherapy, resumption of menses was more likely in subjects using triptorelin with chemotherapy (49.6% vs 63.3%; 95% confidence interval, 1.0%–26.5%; P = .03). The investigators calculated that 6 patients needed to be treated with GnRHa to prevent 1 from persistent amenorrhea.[74] A meta-analysis of 6 randomized trials concluded in favor of GnRHa cotreatment with higher rates of spontaneous resumption of menses and ovulation. However, there was no demonstrable improvement in pregnancy rate.[72] Similarly, another recent meta-analysis of 12 randomized and nonrandomized studies of women with breast cancer demonstrated no benefit in fertility preservation by using GnRHa gonadal protection.[75]

Although controversial, in children or young women with cancer, some experts recommend the use of GnRHa gonadal protection with initial chemotherapy to increase the probability of retaining ovulation and ovarian function. However, there is no present evidence that this modality will preserve fertility. Affected young women and men should be counseled at the time of diagnosis about other fertility preservation methods, such as gamete cryopreservation, even if they display ambivalence.

PSYCHOLOGICAL CONSEQUENCES OF FERTILITY PRESERVATION: MALES

For more than 70 years, sperm cryopreservation has been used as a mechanism to preserve fertility. This intervention has become even more practical and effective with the development of IVF via intracytoplasmic sperm injection. As the use of fertility preservation has increased among at-risk populations (including those diagnosed with cancer), so have the considerations regarding the effects that banking may have on quality-of-life outcomes, including psychological functioning. Men who are younger, more educated, and/or childless are most likely to bank sperm, whereas those with all their desired children or a history of infertility/vasectomy are less likely to bank.[76,77] Regardless, fertility preservation in adult men is often associated with a sense of peace and hopefulness for the future even during the period of impending cancer therapy.[78–80] Of adult males, 96% would recommend sperm banking to other patients, and banking has been associated with significant psychological relief even if the sample is never used.[81] In contrast, those who do not bank and are suspected to have infertility commonly report conflict within intimate relationships, risky sexual behavior, lower self-esteem, and concerns about being rejected by future partners.[82,83] Fertility-related distress is a long-term issue that can impair quality of life for many years after treatment, and banking is one intervention that appears to improve associated psychological outcomes.[84]

Although sperm banking has become a more common practice among adults, much less is known about fertility preservation among adolescents. Adolescents are less likely to bank than adults; and it appears that higher Tanner stage, history of masturbation, perceptions of fertility risk, communication of fertility risk, recommendations to bank by providers and parents, higher banking self-efficacy, beneficial perceptions of banking, higher socioeconomic status, being diagnosed with a nonleukemia/lymphoma, and self-identifying as nonevangelical all associate (on the univariate level) with banking/attempting to bank sperm among adolescents newly diagnosed with cancer.[85,86] Ginsberg and colleagues[87] reported that 55% of adolescents and 88% of their parents had favorable initial impression of sperm banking, and that most families reported that the timing of sperm banking communications had been acceptable. One hundred percent of patients and parents responded "Yes" to the question "Did you make the right decision to attempt banking?" including those adolescents who attempted to bank but failed. Finally, 20% of the sample had to delay treatment to bank, but all of these families felt that banking was worth the delay. Finally, adolescents newly diagnosed with cancer were more likely than their mothers and fathers to prioritize fertility as a "top 3" life goal (behind good future health and work/school success), with youths ranking fertility as being significantly more important than future home ownership or financial wealth.[88]

PSYCHOLOGICAL CONSEQUENCES OF FERTILITY PRESERVATION: FEMALES

Whereas 18% to 31% of at-risk male patients cryopreserve sperm before potentially sterilizing cancer therapy, only 2% to 12% of female patients with similar threats engage in fertility preservation.[76,79,85,89,90] Preservation rates may be lower in female patients as embryo cryopreservation is typically used by women in current partnerships. As oocyte cryopreservation was recognized as a safe and effective fertility preservation method by the American Society of Reproductive Medicine only in October of 2012, rates of utilization for this intervention are even lower. Although several experimental fertility preservation methods may be offered, embryo and oocyte cryopreservation are among the few clinically accepted interventions available for female patients at this time to preserve fertility potential. Ruddy and colleagues[90] recently reported that 11.6% (72/620) of women within a multicenter cohort study for early-stage breast cancer used fertility preservation with 46 (7%) using embryo cryopreservation, 7 (1%) using oocyte cryopreservation, and 19 (3%) using an experimental GnRHa intervention. Interestingly, the proportion of women who used fertility preservation in this study significantly increased from 5% in 2005 to 15% in 2012. An additional 117 (19%) of these women chose alternative cancer therapies (ranging from refusal of endocrine therapy to choosing one chemotherapy regimen over another) to reduce the likelihood of treatment-related infertility. Psychologically speaking, women are more likely to experience fertility-related distress than men, with risk factors such as history of chemotherapy, younger age, being non-White, and/or being childless placing women at highest risk.[90–92]

Less is known about fertility preservation in adolescent girls diagnosed with cancer, as the options available to this subgroup have traditionally been extremely limited. Burns and colleagues[93] examined interests in fertility preservation (along with willingness to wait ≥ 1 month to start therapy) among adolescent girls on treatment for childhood cancer and their parents. Among participating families, most adolescents (80.6%) and their parents (93.1%) endorsed interest in oocyte preservation, but only 29% of adolescents and 19.2% of parents were theoretically willing to delay treatment to complete this process.[93] As ovarian stimulation and subsequent egg harvesting can now take as few as 10 to 14 days, this intervention is now being offered clinically to adolescent girls. Wallace and colleagues[94] recently reported that 21 of 34 families with young daughters at risk for premature ovarian insufficiency (aged 1.2–16.4 years) consented to ovarian tissue cryopreservation, a technique that remains experimental. Regardless of actual risk, parents with children diagnosed with cancer are concerned about potential infertility and are willing to pursue fertility preservation, even within an experimental context.[95]

SUMMARY

Strategies used to accomplish fertility preservation are many. Over the past several decades, new technologies, especially related to ART and IVF, have greatly expanded ways to accomplish fertility preservation. These advances also have grown the indications for pursing fertility potential in general. Surely, such advances will continue to be optimized in the future. By all indicators, the role for fertility preservation in society and medicine is likely to only increase over the next several decades.

REFERENCES

1. Bunge RG, Sherman JK. Fertilizing capacity of frozen human spermatozoa. Nature 1953;172(4382):767–8.
2. Katz DJ, Kolon TF, Feldman DR, et al. Fertility preservation strategies for male patients with cancer. Nat Rev Urol 2013;10(8):463–72.
3. Wang JH, Muller CH, Lin K. Optimizing fertility preservation for pre- and postpubertal males with cancer. Semin Reprod Med 2013;31(4):274–85.
4. Feldschuh J, Brassel J, Durso N, et al. Successful sperm storage for 28 years. Fertil Steril 2005;84(4):1017.
5. Paoli D, Lombardo F, Lenzi A, et al. Sperm cryopreservation: effects on chromatin structure. Adv Exp Med Biol 2014;791:137–50.
6. Williams DH 4th. Fertility preservation in the male with cancer. Curr Urol Rep 2013;14(4):315–26.
7. Loren AW, Mangu PB, Beck LN, et al. Fertility preservation for patients with cancer: American Society of Clinical Oncology clinical practice guideline update. J Clin Oncol 2013;31(19):2500–10.
8. Pastuszak AW, Lai WS, Hsieh TC, et al. Posthumous sperm utilization in men presenting for sperm banking: an analysis of patient choice. Andrology 2013;1(2):251–5.
9. Klock S. A survey of sperm donors' attitudes: a much-needed perspective. Fertil Steril 2014;101(1):43–4.
10. Steptoe PC, Edwards RG. Birth after the reimplantation of a human embryo. Lancet 1978;2(8085):366.
11. Zhao Y, Brezina P, Hsu CC, et al. In vitro fertilization: four decades of reflections and promises. Biochim Biophys Acta 2011;1810(9):843–52.
12. Konc J, Kanyo K, Kriston R, et al. Cryopreservation of embryos and oocytes in human assisted reproduction. Biomed Res Int 2014;2014:307268.
13. Nagy ZP, Chang CC, Shapiro DB, et al. The efficacy and safety of human oocyte vitrification. Semin Reprod Med 2009;27(6):450–5.

14. Willadsen S, Polge C, Rowson LE. The viability of deep-frozen cow embryos. J Reprod Fertil 1978;52(2):391–3.
15. Mukaida T, Nakamura S, Tomiyama T, et al. Successful birth after transfer of vitrified human blastocysts with use of a cryoloop containerless technique. Fertil Steril 2001;76(3):618–20.
16. Arav A. Cryopreservation of oocytes and embryos. Theriogenology 2014;81(1): 96–102.
17. Vajta G, Nagy ZP, Cobo A, et al. Vitrification in assisted reproduction: myths, mistakes, disbeliefs and confusion. Reprod Biomed Online 2009;19(Suppl 3):1–7.
18. Cil AP, Seli E. Current trends and progress in clinical applications of oocyte cryopreservation. Curr Opin Obstet Gynecol 2013;25(3):247–54.
19. Potdar N, Gelbaya TA, Nardo LG. Oocyte vitrification in the 21st century and post-warming fertility outcomes: a systematic review and meta-analysis. Reprod Biomed Online 2014;29(2):159–76.
20. Wong KM, Mastenbroek S, Repping S. Cryopreservation of human embryos and its contribution to in vitro fertilization success rates. Fertil Steril 2014;102(1):19–26.
21. Fabbri R, Porcu E, Marsella T, et al. Technical aspects of oocyte cryopreservation. Mol Cell Endocrinol 2000;169(1–2):39–42.
22. Nagy ZP, Nel-Themaat L, Chang CC, et al. Cryopreservation of eggs. Methods Mol Biol 2014;1154:439–54.
23. Practice Committees of American Society for Reproductive Medicine, Society for Assisted Reproductive Technology. Mature oocyte cryopreservation: a guideline. Fertil Steril 2013;99(1):37–43.
24. ACOG: Committee opinion no. 584: oocyte cryopreservation. Obstet Gynecol 2014;123(1):221–2.
25. Brezina PR, Ke RW, Ding J, et al. The impact of elective egg freezing technology. J IVF Reprod Med Genet 2013;1:e103.
26. United States Census Bureau. The 2006 statistical abstract. 2006. Available at: https://www.census.gov/compendia/statab/2006/2006edition.html. Accessed September 1, 2014.
27. Health Improvement Scotland long term follow up of survivors of childhood cancer. A national clinical guideline. 2013. Available at: http://www.sign.ac.uk/pdf/sign132.pdf. Accessed September 1, 2014.
28. Barton SE, Najita JS, Ginsburg ES, et al. Infertility, infertility treatment, and achievement of pregnancy in female survivors of childhood cancer: a report from the Childhood Cancer Survivor Study cohort. Lancet Oncol 2013;14(9):873–81.
29. Committee opinion no. 605: primary ovarian insufficiency in adolescents and young women. Obstet Gynecol 2014;124(1):193–7.
30. Roness H, Kalich-Philosoph L, Meirow D. Prevention of chemotherapy-induced ovarian damage: possible roles for hormonal and non-hormonal attenuating agents. Hum Reprod Update 2014;20(5):759–74.
31. Practice Committee of American Society for Reproductive Medicine. Fertility preservation in patients undergoing gonadotoxic therapy or gonadectomy: a committee opinion. Fertil Steril 2013;100(5):1214–23.
32. Ethics Committee of American Society for Reproductive Medicine. Fertility preservation and reproduction in patients facing gonadotoxic therapies: a committee opinion. Fertil Steril 2013,100(5):1224–31.
33. Mills M, Rindfuss RR, McDonald P, et al. Why do people postpone parenthood? Reasons and social policy incentives. Hum Reprod Update 2011;17(6):848–60.
34. Cobo A, Diaz C. Clinical application of oocyte vitrification: a systematic review and meta-analysis of randomized controlled trials. Fertil Steril 2011;96(2):277–85.

35. Gook DA, Edgar DH. Human oocyte cryopreservation. Hum Reprod Update 2007;13(6):591–605.
36. Chen C. Pregnancy after human oocyte cryopreservation. Lancet 1986;1(8486): 884–6.
37. Oktay K, Cil AP, Bang H. Efficiency of oocyte cryopreservation: a meta-analysis. Fertil Steril 2006;86(1):70–80.
38. Rienzi L, Romano S, Albricci L, et al. Embryo development of fresh 'versus' vitrified metaphase II oocytes after ICSI: a prospective randomized sibling-oocyte study. Hum Reprod 2010;25(1):66–73.
39. Borini A, Levi Setti PE, Anserini P, et al. Multicenter observational study on slow-cooling oocyte cryopreservation: clinical outcome. Fertil Steril 2010;94(5):1662–8.
40. Brannstrom M, Diaz-Garcia C. Transplantation of female genital organs. J Obstet Gynaecol Res 2011;37(4):271–91.
41. Meirow D. Reproduction post-chemotherapy in young cancer patients. Mol Cell Endocrinol 2000;169(1–2):123–31.
42. Anchan RM, Ginsburg ES. Fertility concerns and preservation in younger women with breast cancer. Crit Rev Oncol Hematol 2010;74(3):175–92.
43. Oktem O, Urman B. Options of fertility preservation in female cancer patients. Obstet Gynecol Surv 2010;65(8):531–42.
44. Wallace WH, Thomson AB, Kelsey TW. The radiosensitivity of the human oocyte. Hum Reprod 2003;18(1):117–21.
45. Paris F, Perez GI, Fuks Z, et al. Sphingosine 1-phosphate preserves fertility in irradiated female mice without propagating genomic damage in offspring. Nat Med 2002;8(9):901–2.
46. Wallace WH, Thomson AB, Saran F, et al. Predicting age of ovarian failure after radiation to a field that includes the ovaries. Int J Radiat Oncol Biol Phys 2005; 62(3):738–44.
47. Wallace WH, Anderson RA, Irvine DS. Fertility preservation for young patients with cancer: who is at risk and what can be offered? Lancet Oncol 2005;6(4):209–18.
48. Elizur SE, Tulandi T, Meterissian S, et al. Fertility preservation for young women with rectal cancer–a combined approach from one referral center. J Gastrointest Surg 2009;13(6):1111–5.
49. Noyes N, Knopman JM, Long K, et al. Fertility considerations in the management of gynecologic malignancies. Gynecol Oncol 2011;120(3):326–33.
50. Williams RS, Littell RD, Mendenhall NP. Laparoscopic oophoropexy and ovarian function in the treatment of Hodgkin disease. Cancer 1999;86(10):2138–42.
51. Husseinzadeh N, Nahhas WA, Velkley DE, et al. The preservation of ovarian function in young women undergoing pelvic radiation therapy. Gynecol Oncol 1984; 18(3):373–9.
52. Terenziani M, Piva L, Meazza C, et al. Oophoropexy: a relevant role in preservation of ovarian function after pelvic irradiation. Fertil Steril 2009;91(3):935.e15–6.
53. Jenninga E, Hilders CG, Louwe LA, et al. Female fertility preservation: practical and ethical considerations of an underused procedure. Cancer J 2008;14(5):333–9.
54. Clough KB, Goffinet F, Labib A, et al. Laparoscopic unilateral ovarian transposition prior to irradiation: prospective study of 20 cases. Cancer 1996;77(12):2638–45.
55. Damewood MD, Hesla HS, Lowen M, et al. Induction of ovulation and pregnancy following lateral oophoropexy for Hodgkin's disease. Int J Gynaecol Obstet 1990; 33(4):369–71.
56. Zinger M, Liu JH, Husseinzadeh N, et al. Successful surrogate pregnancy after ovarian transposition, pelvic irradiation and hysterectomy. J Reprod Med 2004; 49(7):573–4.

57. Blumenfeld Z. Ovarian rescue/protection from chemotherapeutic agents. J Soc Gynecol Investig 2001;8(1 Suppl Proceedings):S60–4.
58. Buekers TE, Anderson B, Sorosky JI, et al. Ovarian function after surgical treatment for cervical cancer. Gynecol Oncol 2001;80(1):85–8.
59. Pfeifer SM, Coutifaris C. Reproductive technologies 1998: options available for the cancer patient. Med Pediatr Oncol 1999;33(1):34–40.
60. Morice P, Thiam-Ba R, Castaigne D, et al. Fertility results after ovarian transposition for pelvic malignancies treated by external irradiation or brachytherapy. Hum Reprod 1998;13(3):660–3.
61. Barton SE, Politch JA, Benson CB, et al. Transabdominal follicular aspiration for oocyte retrieval in patients with ovaries inaccessible by transvaginal ultrasound. Fertil Steril 2011;95(5):1773–6.
62. Lee SJ, Schover LR, Partridge AH, et al. American Society of Clinical Oncology recommendations on fertility preservation in cancer patients. J Clin Oncol 2006;24(18):2917–31.
63. Fageeh W, Raffa H, Jabbad H, et al. Transplantation of the human uterus. Int J Gynaecol Obstet 2002;76(3):245–51.
64. World's first successful uterus transplant performed in Turkey. 2011. Available at: http://rt.com/news/first-uterus-surgery-success-845/. Accessed August 29, 2014.
65. Womb transplant recipient Derya Sert pregnant. Available at: http://www.news.com.au/technology/science/womb-transplant-recipient-derya-sert-pregnant/story-fn5fsgyc-1226619553524. Accessed August 29, 2014.
66. Nine Swedish women undergo uterus transplants. Available at: http://www.cbsnews.com/news/nine-swedish-women-undergo-uterus-transplants/. Accessed August 29, 2014.
67. Eraslan S, Hamernik RJ, Hardy JD. Replantation of uterus and ovaries in dogs, with successful pregnancy. Arch Surg 1966;92(1):9–12.
68. Truta E, Pop I, Popa D, et al. Experimental re- and transplantation of the internal female genital organs. Rom Med Rev 1969;13(1):53–8.
69. Barzilai A, Paldi E, Gal D, et al. Autotransplantation of the uterus and ovaries in dogs. Isr J Med Sci 1973;9(1):49–52.
70. Racho El-Akouri R, Kurlberg G, Dindelegan G, et al. Heterotopic uterine transplantation by vascular anastomosis in the mouse. J Endocrinol 2002;174(2):157–66.
71. Wranning CA, Marcickiewicz J, Enskog A, et al. Fertility after autologous ovine uterine-tubal-ovarian transplantation by vascular anastomosis to the external iliac vessels. Hum Reprod 2010;25(8):1973–9.
72. Bedaiwy MA, Abou-Setta AM, Desai N, et al. Gonadotropin-releasing hormone analog cotreatment for preservation of ovarian function during gonadotoxic chemotherapy: a systematic review and meta-analysis. Fertil Steril 2011;95(3):906–14.e1-4.
73. Meirow D, Epstein M, Lewis H, et al. Administration of cyclophosphamide at different stages of follicular maturation in mice: effects on reproductive performance and fetal malformations. Hum Reprod 2001;16(4):632–7.
74. Del Mastro L, Boni L, Michelotti A, et al. Effect of the gonadotropin-releasing hormone analogue triptorelin on the occurrence of chemotherapy-induced early menopause in premenopausal women with breast cancer: a randomized trial. JAMA 2011;306(3):269–76.
75. Turnor NH, Partridge A, Sanna G, et al. Utility of gonadotropin-releasing hormone agonists for fertility preservation in young breast cancer patients: the benefit remains uncertain. Ann Oncol 2013;24(9):2224–35.
76. Girasole CR, Cookson MS, Smith JA Jr, et al. Sperm banking: use and outcomes in patients treated for testicular cancer. BJU Int 2007;99(1):33–6.

77. Schover LR, Brey K, Lichtin A, et al. Knowledge and experience regarding cancer, infertility, and sperm banking in younger male survivors. J Clin Oncol 2002; 20(7):1880–9.
78. Pacey A. Sperm you can bank on. Br J Cancer 2003;327.
79. Pacey A, Merrick H, Arden-Close E, et al. Implications of sperm banking for health-related quality of life up to 1 year after cancer diagnosis. Br J Cancer 2013;108(5): 1004–11.
80. Pacey AA, Eiser C. Banking sperm is only the first of many decisions for men: what healthcare professionals and men need to know. Hum Fertil 2011;14(4): 208–17.
81. Saito K, Suzuki K, Iwasaki A, et al. Sperm cryopreservation before cancer chemotherapy helps in the emotional battle against cancer. Cancer 2005;104(3):521–4.
82. Chapple A, Salinas M, Ziebland S, et al. Fertility issues: the perceptions and experiences of young men recently diagnosed and treated for cancer. J Adolesc Health 2007;40(1):69–75.
83. Zebrack BJ, Casillas J, Nohr L, et al. Fertility issues for young adult survivors of childhood cancer. Psychooncology 2004;13(10):689–99.
84. Hammond C, Abrams JR, Syrjala KL. Fertility and risk factors for elevated infertility concern in 10-year hematopoietic cell transplant survivors and case-matched controls. J Clin Oncol 2007;25(23):3511–7.
85. Klosky JL, Randolph ME, Navid F, et al. Sperm cryopreservation practices among adolescent cancer patients at risk for infertility. Pediatr Hematol Oncol 2009; 26(4):252–60.
86. Klosky JL, Russell KM, Zhang H, et al. Adolescent sperm banking in North America: results from the sbank10 study. Fertil Steril 2014;102(3 Supplement):e159.
87. Ginsberg JP, Ogle SK, Tuchman LK, et al. Sperm banking for adolescent and young adult cancer patients: sperm quality, patient, and parent perspectives. Pediatr Blood Cancer 2008;50(3):594–8.
88. Klosky JL, Simmons JL, Russell KM, et al. Fertility as a priority among at-risk adolescent males newly diagnosed with cancer and their parents. Support Care Cancer 2014. [Epub ahead of print].
89. Armuand GM, Rodriguez-Wallberg KA, Wettergren L, et al. Sex differences in fertility-related information received by young adult cancer survivors. J Clin Oncol 2012;30(17):2147–53.
90. Ruddy KJ, Gelber SI, Tamimi RM, et al. Prospective study of fertility concerns and preservation strategies in young women with breast cancer. J Clin Oncol 2014; 32(11):1151–6.
91. Canada AL, Schover LR. The psychosocial impact of interrupted childbearing in long-term female cancer survivors. Psychooncology 2012;21(2):134–43.
92. Geue K, Richter D, Schmidt R, et al. The desire for children and fertility issues among young German cancer survivors. J Adolesc Health 2014;54(5):527–35.
93. Burns KC, Boudreau C, Panepinto JA. Attitudes regarding fertility preservation in female adolescent cancer patients. J Pediatr Hematol Oncol 2006;28(6):350–4.
94. Wallace WH, Smith AG, Kelsey TW, et al. Fertility preservation for girls and young women with cancer: population-based validation of criteria for ovarian tissue cryopreservation. Lancet Oncol 2014;15(10):1129–36.
95. Oosterhuis BE, Goodwin T, Kiernan M, et al. Concerns about infertility risks among pediatric oncology patients and their parents. Pediatr Blood Cancer 2008;50(1):85–9.

Endocrine and Reproductive Effects of Polycystic Ovarian Syndrome

Laura C. Ecklund, MD[a], Rebecca S. Usadi, MD[b],*

KEYWORDS

- Polycystic ovary syndrome • Reproductive endocrinology • Clomiphene citrate
- Letrozole • Live birth rate • Infertility

KEY POINTS

- Polycystic ovarian syndrome (PCOS) is defined by hyperandrogenism, ovulatory dysfunction, and polycystic ovaries on ultrasonography.
- Weight loss should be encouraged for overweight and obese women with PCOS.
- Combined oral contraceptive pills remain the first-line treatment of hyperandrogenism in women not seeking pregnancy.
- Metformin is no longer indicated as a primary ovulation induction agent.
- Letrozole was found to have higher live birth and ovulation rates in women with PCOS compared with clomiphene in a recent multicenter, randomized trial.

INTRODUCTION

Polycystic ovarian syndrome (PCOS) is the most common cause of ovulatory dysfunction in women. Although the clinical expression varies widely, the syndrome is classically described by hyperandrogenism, ovulatory dysfunction, and polycystic ovaries. PCOS occurs in 5% to 15% of women, depending on which diagnostic criteria are used.[1] There is a considerable multisystem impact of this disorder that spans from systemic metabolic disturbances to reproductive difficulty to long-term cardiovascular health and cancer risk. The effect of PCOS on endocrine and menstrual function, fertility, and reproductive outcome and the management of these sequelae are discussed in this review.

The diagnostic criteria for PCOS vary depending on different expert groups. It is generally accepted that PCOS is defined as hyperandrogenism and ovulatory

The authors declare no conflicts of interest and no funding support.
[a] Carolinas Medical Center, 1000 Blythe Boulevard, Charlotte, NC 28203, USA; [b] Reproductive Endocrinology and Infertility, Carolinas Medical Center, 1000 Blythe Boulevard, Charlotte, NC 28203, USA
* Corresponding author.
E-mail address: Rebecca.Usadi@carolinashealthcare.org

dysfunction. The commonly used 2003 Rotterdam criteria added ultrasonographic findings of ovarian appearance to the diagnosis. To meet the Rotterdam Consensus criteria, 2 of the 3 features need to be documented.[2] Hyperandrogenism may be diagnosed from clinical findings or by serum testosterone concentrations. Two common clinical signs of hyperandrogenism are hirsutism and acne. Polycystic ovaries are sonographically diagnosed by the presence of 12 or more antral follicles, measuring 2 to 9 mm in diameter, or increased ovarian volume greater than 10 cm³ on either ovary.[2] Fundamental to the diagnosis of PCOS is the exclusion of other potential causes of the clinical or biochemical findings. The most common endocrinopathies to rule out are thyroid dysfunction and hyperprolactinemia. Less common disorders that may mimic symptoms of PCOS include nonclassic congenital adrenal hyperplasia, Cushing syndrome, androgen-secreting neoplasms, or acromegaly.[3]

The etiology of PCOS remains unclear and is likely multifactorial. Prenatal exposure to testosterone and genetic, and epigenetic effects have been implicated. Insulin resistance is believed to play a significant role, particularly in overweight and obese patients with PCOS. Increased levels of insulin cause decreased amounts of sex hormone binding globulin (SHBG), which, in turn, leads to increased amounts of free circulating androgens.[2]

MENSTRUAL AND ENDOMETRIAL EFFECTS

Oligomenorrhea and secondary amenorrhea are common presenting symptoms among patients with PCOS. Women with amenorrhea have been found to have increased metabolic risk with severe hyperandrogenism and higher antral follicle counts.[1] Although information about spontaneous ovulation rates in women with PCOS is limited, a large randomized controlled trial reported ovulation in up to 32% of cycles.[4] Correctly recognizing PCOS in adolescent females with oligomenorrhea is more difficult than in adults. This difficulty arises because most menstrual cycles are anovulatory during the first 3 years after menarche.[5] Adolescents also commonly have acne and often have high antral follicle counts on sonographic measurement. Given the complexity of diagnosing PCOS in adolescent females, the Endocrine Society has suggested specific diagnostic criteria. In contrast to adults, in whom only 2 of the 3 Rotterdam criteria are necessary to make a diagnosis, adolescents require all 3 elements to confirm the diagnosis, based on the Endocrine Society suggestions. Oligomenorrhea or amenorrhea should be present for at least 2 years after menarche in these females. Primary amenorrhea after the age of 16 years also satisfies the diagnostic criteria. The sonographic findings must include an ovarian volume of greater than 10 cm³, because polycystic ovaries are a common finding among adolescent girls. Hyperandrogenism must be diagnosed by increased androgen levels, because acne is often a common finding among adolescents.

Menstrual irregularity is not without risk. Women with PCOS are exposed to prolonged amounts of unopposed estrogen, and a relationship between PCOS and endometrial cancer has been described. The severity of oligo-ovulation may correlate with endometrial thickness and subsequent endometrial hyperplasia in women. When comparing aged-matched women with and without PCOS, proliferative endometrium was observed significantly more often in the PCOS group. Data support a 2.7-fold increased risk of endometrial cancer in women with PCOS.[6] It has been suggested that women have a minimum of 4 withdrawal bleeds per year and undergo potential surveillance measures to reduce the risk of endometrial hyperplasia.[1] These measures could include endometrial biopsy or ultrasonography to assess endometrial thickening for women with expended periods of amenorrhea. According to the American College of Obstetricians and Gynecologists (ACOG) recommendations for management of abnormal uterine bleeding associated with ovulatory dysfunction, women aged 19 to 39 years who fail medical treatment or have prolonged exposure to unopposed estrogen are candidates for endometrial assessment with biopsy. Furthermore, all women older than 45 years with anovulatory bleeding are candidates for endometrial biopsy.[7]

Current recommended treatments for PCOS focus on controlling weight, hormone balance, and insulin resistance. Obesity contributes considerably to the reproductive and metabolic abnormalities in women with PCOS. Obesity increases the risk of metabolic syndrome, diabetes mellitus, insulin resistance, and dyslipidemia. The prevalence of obesity in women with PCOS varies widely across different geographic regions, from 10% in Italy to up to 76% in the United States and Australia.[1] Body fat distribution in PCOS tends to have a centripetal distribution. Greater abdominal adiposity is associated with greater insulin resistance.[1] Several studies have shown that weight loss can decrease circulating androgen levels, improve glucose and lipid levels, decrease hirsutism, lead to spontaneous resumption of menses, and improve pregnancy rates.[3] Weight loss, through pharmacologic weight loss agents and gastric bypass surgery, has also shown improvements in menstrual function.[8] Agents such as orlistat, an intestinal inhibitor of lipid absorption, or sibutramine, an anorexic agent, have shown improvement in ovarian function with increased pregnancy rates, decreased hirsutism, and decreased glucose and lipid levels.[9] In this small study, orlistat was effective at weight loss.[9] Weight loss as little as 5% of total body weight has been shown to cause near normalization of reproductive and metabolic abnormalities in several studies.[2]

Hormonal contraception is the current first-line management option for women with PCOS who do not desire pregnancy to help improve menstrual cyclicity. Combination low-dose hormonal contraceptives are the most frequently used. The progestin component suppresses luteinizing hormone levels, which, in turn suppress ovarian androgen production. Some progestins also have antiandrogenic properties and act through antagonizing effects on androgen receptors or inhibit 5-α reductase activity.[2] The estrogen component increases SHBG, which reduces the circulating bioavailable androgens. Although the estrogenic fraction of hormonal contraceptives remains similar between different pills, the progestins differ in their androgenic potential. More androgenic progestins include norethindrone, norgestrel, and levonorgestrel, whereas desogestrel, norgestimate, and gestodene are less androgenic. There are also antiandrogenic progestins, such as drospirenone. In comparison trials of the different progestins, a significant difference in testosterone levels has not been shown.[10] There is evidence that extended cycle hormonal contraceptives provide greater hormonal suppression and prevent rebound ovarian function.[3] Progestin-only hormonal contraceptive pills or intrauterine devices are alternative methods for endometrial protection. However, these methods have been associated with abnormal bleeding patterns and do not have the benefit of increasing SHBG.[2]

Insulin resistance is a common finding in PCOS, and diabetic pharmaceuticals have been used in treatment of this syndrome. Pharmacologic improvement of peripheral insulin sensitivity has been the focus. Biguanides and thiazolidinediones have been studied for their risk/benefit ratio in treating PCOS. Biguanides, like metformin, have been associated with some weight loss and an improvement in menstrual cyclicity and ovulation rate. Metformin is recommended for prevention of diabetes in women with PCOS and impaired glucose tolerance when lifestyle modification is not successful. However, metformin was less effective than oral contraceptive pills (OCPs), in improving menses and reducing serum androgens.[11] Thiazolidinediones, such as pioglitazone, have increased rates of liver toxicity and are pregnancy category C status and therefore no longer commonly used to treat women with PCOS, particularly those trying to conceive. The most recent recommendation is not to screen for insulin resistance, but rather to screen for metabolic syndrome. There is insufficient evidence to recommend prophylactic use of insulin sensitizing agents to prevent diabetes mellitus in women with PCOS.[2] Metformin can be used as a second-line agent for menstrual regulation in women who cannot tolerate or who have contraindications to OCPs.

Women with PCOS often have increased levels of triglycerides, low-density lipoprotein, and non–high-density lipoprotein–cholesterol as well as decreased levels of high-density liproprotein.[3] Statins have been evaluated for their role in PCOS treatment, given these known trends in cholesterol levels. Although appropriate for dyslipidemia, data from a meta-analysis looking at use of statins for PCOS and not specifically weight loss have shown that statins do not improve menstrual cyclicity, ovulation, hirsutism, or acne.[12]

HYPERANDROGENISM

The cutaneous manifestations of PCOS include hirsutism, acne, androgenic alopecia, acanthosis nigricans, and skin tags. Perhaps the best marker of hyperandrogenism is hirsutism. Hirsutism is present in 70% of clinically hyperandrogenic women with PCOS.[13,14] The degree of hirsutism is quantified by the modified Ferriman-Gallwey score, which looks at hair growth in 9 body locations.[13] It tends to be more severe in women with central obesity and may correlate with severity of metabolic sequelae of the disorder. Hirsutism presents when androgens change normally vellous hair to terminal hair in androgen-sensitive areas, most commonly, on facial areas. Terminal hair is pigmented, coarse hair. Treatment is focused on decreasing production and amount of circulating androgens. This treatment is established by inhibiting ovarian androgen synthesis with hormonal contraceptives. The hormonal contraceptives increase SHBG, which decreases bioavailable testosterone. Terminal hair turnover is slow, so the treatment should be continued for at least 6 months before a result can be expected.[15] Antiandrogen treatment includes agents such as spironolactone, an aldosterone antagonist, flutamide, an androgen receptor antagonist, and finasteride, a 5-α reductase type 2 inhibitor. These agents prevent new terminal hair growth but must be used in combination with contraception, given their fetal toxicity. Flutamide is limited by its hepatotoxic nature.[15] Another drug, eflornithine, is the only topical pharmaceutical that has been shown to slow facial hair growth. Its mechanism of action involves irreversibly binding to ornithine decarboxylase, thus preventing the natural substrate from binding its active site.[2,16] Eflornithine was originally developed for cancer treatment, and was found to improve hirsutism in patients who used it. In clinical studies, women treated with eflornithine showed significant clinical improvement over 1 year of use.[16] Insulin sensitizers, like metformin, or thiazolidinedione medications have little effect on hirsutism. Other treatment options include electrolysis and laser treatment.

Acne is another common cutaneous manifestation of PCOS, although it is not as suggestive of hyperandrogenism as hirsutism. Isolated acne and alopecia are not good indicators of hyperandrogenism. Increased androgens increase sebum production within the pilosebaceous unit. The sebum accumulates, and together with desquamated follicular cells and *Propionibacterium acnes* bacteria, creates comedones.[17] Although largely focused on the face of individuals with PCOS, acne may also be located on the neck, chest, and upper back.[18] Medications that decrease free circulating androgens, like hormonal contraceptives, may be used as appropriate treatment of acne. Severe acne can be treated with isotrentoin, although this may simultaneously cause alopecia. Insulin sensitizers are not recommended for treatment of acne, because they are less effective for this indication than OCPs. Combined OCPs remain the first-line treatment of hyperandrogenism and many are approved by the US Food and Drug Administration (FDA) for the treatment of acne and hirsutism.[19] The mechanism of action for OCPs is the inhibition of ovarian steroid production with estrogen and progestin. Spironolactone has been used for its antiandrogen effect in combination with OCPs to block androgen action at the hair follicles.[19] Given the potential of spironolactone to cause teratogenic effects in a fetus, it should not be used without OCPs.

Androgenic alopecia is a less frequent cutaneous manifestation of PCOS and may present later in the disease course. Alopecia is terminal hair loss, largely at the scalp of females with PCOS.[20] There is a poor correlation between alopecia and biochemical hyperandrogenism, unless present with oligomenorrhea.[21] However, an association between alopecia, metabolic syndrome, and insulin resistance has been described. Pathophysiology of alopecia with hyperandrogenism centers on decreased aromatase activity and androgen receptor overexpression in balding areas.[22]

INFERTILITY

Women with PCOS are often subfertile secondary to ovulatory dysfunction, problems with oocyte quality, and endometrial receptivity. Associations have been made between obesity and oligomenorrhea with decreased fecundity. Increasing abdominal obesity with subsequent increased insulin resistance exacerbates reproductive abnormalities. Increased ovarian hyperandrogenism and hyperinsulinemia cause premature granulosa cell luteinization and disruption of the intrafollicular environment, leading to impaired oocyte maturation.[1] Impaired insulin signaling and glucose metabolism lead to impaired oocyte metabolism.[1] Body mass index (BMI, calculated as weight in kilograms divided by the square of height in meters) is positively associated with levels of total and free testosterone and SHBG. Studies have shown a dose-response relationship with reproductive abnormalities and BMI. The PPCOS II (Pregnancy in Polycystic Ovarian Syndrome II) trial showed increased time from randomization to live birth with increasing BMI.[23]

The primary treatment of anovulatory infertility in PCOS is weight loss through lifestyle modification. There is evidence for increased pregnancy rate and decreased requirement for ovulation induction agents in small controlled trials with weight reduction. Menstrual function was shown to be improved with as little as 5% to 10% reduction in total body weight in a small but often cited study.[24] No one diet has proved to be more beneficial than others. The important factor is calorie restriction. Studies have shown no significant difference in outcomes between different hypocaloric diets.[25]

Clomiphene citrate has been the first-line treatment of ovulation induction in women with PCOS since its FDA approval in the 1960s. Clomiphene is a selective estrogen receptor modulator, which acts on the hypothalamus to inhibit the negative feedback of circulating estrogen. This inhibition leads to increased ovarian stimulation by endogenous gonadotropins, thereby stimulating follicular development.[23] Clomiphene citrate is not without its limitations, including poor overall success rate, concern for multifetal gestation, ovarian hyperstimulation syndrome (OHSS), pelvic pain, and vasomotor symptoms. Research has shown a 23% live birth rate when using clomiphene as an ovulation induction agent.[26] Multifetal gestation is as high as 4% to 8% with this method.[23] The PPCOS I (Pregnancy in Polycystic Ovarian Syndrome I) trial explored using extended release metformin alone or with clomiphene for ovulation induction. In this study, clomiphene was found to be 3 times more effective than metformin at achieving live birth rates.[23] The indications for metformin in PCOS are limited, and metformin is no longer recommended as a first-line ovulation induction agent based on this trial. This recommendation is further supported by a meta-analysis by the Cochrane Database Systematic Review in 2012, in which there was no evidence that metformin improved live birth rates alone or in combination with clomiphene.[10]

A secondary analysis of this trial examined the use of progestin for a withdrawal bleed before ovarian stimulation. Another practice, called the "stair-step" method of prescribing clomiphene in increasing doses without inducing a withdrawal bleed in the woman has not had an ovulatory response to the lower dose.[27,28] The common clinical practice of inducing endometrial shedding with progestin before ovarian stimulation was found to have an adverse effect on the rate of conception and live birth in anovulatory women with PCOS. In this analysis, 29.8% of conceptions followed spontaneous menses, 8.4% followed anovulatory cycles with progestin withdrawal, and 61.8% followed anovulatory cycles without a progestin-induced withdrawal bleed.[29] This situation may be caused by excessive shedding and inadequate regrowth of the basalis layers in the subsequent cycle. Aromatase inhibitors, such as letrozole, were developed as an adjunctive treatment of breast cancer and act by preventing the conversion of androgens to estrogens. They free the hypothalamic-pituitary axis from excessive estrogen feedback and have been used as an alternative to clomiphene.[26] The benefits of aromatase inhibitors include a lower multiple follicle recruitment rate and decreased multifetal pregnancy rate. PPCOS II reported a higher cumulative live birth rate in women who received letrozole compared with those who received clomiphene (27.5% versus 19.1%), as shown in **Fig. 1**.[23] Limitations of letrozole include the fact that it is a pregnancy category X drug, similar to clomiphene, so appropriate counseling needs to be taken with patients to ensure that they do not inadvertently begin either drug if already pregnant. Several Canadian studies have found no significant fetal teratogenic effects after appropriate letrozole use for ovulation

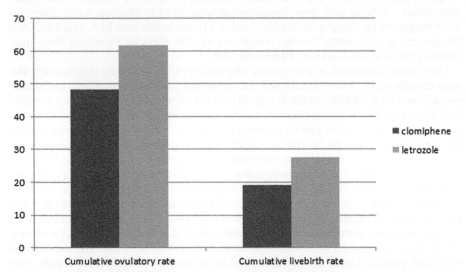

Fig. 1. Letrozole versus clomiphene in measuring ovulatory rate and live birth rate. (*Data from* Legro R, Brzyski R, Diamond M, et al. Letrozole versus clomiphene for infertility in the polycystic ovary syndrome. N Engl J Med 2014;371:119–29.)

induction.[26] In PPCOS II, letrozole was associated with a lower twin pregnancy rate than clomiphene, although this aspect of the study was underpowered to detect a true significant difference. Further trials are needed to explore the evidence that letrozole is superior to clomiphene as a treatment of infertility in women with PCOS.

In women with clomiphene resistance, several adjunctive treatments have been described. Alternative treatment protocols include adding dexamethasone to clomiphene in clomiphene-resistant women. This treatment has been shown, in several studies, to increase ovulation and pregnancy rates.[28] One trial used a high dose of dexamethasone in addition to clomiphene and found higher ovulation rates with the combination than with clomiphene and placebo.[29]

Gonadotropins are also used as ovulation induction agents in women with PCOS. Doses of gonadotropins start at 37.5 IU/d, with gradual increases in dose to stimulate follicular development with the step-up protocol. The step-down protocol begins with a higher loading dose of gonadotropin and progresses with decreasing levels of the drug as follicular development is visualized with ultrasonographic monitoring.[30] Limitations of this type of ovulation induction agent are multifollicular recruitment with subsequent OHSS. OHSS occurs when presence of multiple luteinized cysts within the ovaries cause vascular hyperpermeability, with resulting third spacing of fluids. Women with OHSS may become hypovolemic from fluid shifts with subsequent hemoconcentration, thrombosis, oliguria, pleural effusion, and respiratory distress in the severe form of the syndrome.[1] To avoid this severe outcome, it is recommended to cancel cycles in which there are multifollicular development or documented high estradiol levels.[31] The risk of multifetal gestation is also increased with this method of ovulation induction. One meta-analysis evaluated the effect of metformin in combination with gonadotropins for ovulation induction in women with PCOS.[32] The study found that metformin increases live birth and pregnancy rate in patients with PCOS when used in combination with gonadotropins. This review was limited by several factors and further studies are required to confirm the results.

In vitro fertilization (IVF) remains an option for conception in women with PCOS who do not respond to ovulation induction agents. The Thessaloniki ESHRE/ASRM-Sponsored PCOS Consensus Workshop Group recommended IVF as third-line treatment after step-up gonadotropin protocols, although this needs to be readdressed with the outcome of the recent PPCOS II data.[33] IVF has the advantage of limiting multifetal gestation by using single embryo transfer. However, there remains the risk of OHSS. Several studies have examined the live birth rate in women with and without PCOS who use IVF for fertility treatment. In one retrospective study, the live birth rates after IVF in women with and without PCOS were found to be similar.[34] Further analysis compared live birth rates between women with PCOS who were obese to those women with PCOS who had a BMI less than 30. The results showed an infant take-home rate of one-third in the obese group compared with one-half in the nonobese women.[34] The live birth rate with IVF treatment in women with PCOS declines with increasing BMI. In obese women with PCOS undergoing IVF, the odds of live birth were 71% lower per cycle start than in lean women with PCOS.[35] This finding provides further support for weight loss before IVF treatment in obese women. Metformin has not been shown to improve pregnancy rates with IVF but has shown a reduced rate of severe OHSS.[36] Another method of reducing the risk of severe OHSS in IVF stimulations is use of leuprolide to trigger egg maturation instead of the more commonly used human chorionic gonadotropin. Leuprolide can be used as a gonadotropin-releasing hormone (GnRH) agonist to trigger oocyte maturation after cotreatment with a GnRH antagonist to allow for endogenous gonadotropins to stimulate the final stages of oocyte maturation. The endogenous gonadotropins have a shorter half-life, leading to subsequent earlier luteolysis and decreased risk of OHSS. Further studies are needed with the leuprolide trigger protocol.[31]

Laparoscopic ovarian drilling is an alternative to those women with PCOS who have clomiphene resistance. It is performed with either electrocautery or laser, with electrocautery being the more commonly used method.[37] This procedure is commonly performed by inserting a laparoscopic needle with unipolar ability into the ovarian stroma to induce thermal damage to the underlying tissue. It is the underlying stromal tissue that is responsible for androgen production. Laparoscopic ovarian drilling restores ovulation in about 50% of women with improvement in menstrual regularity.[2] Rates of conception after the procedure are about 50% over the first year. Laparoscopic ovarian drilling has been compared with other medical treatment groups. The live birth rate in one large meta-analysis was not significantly different from other medical treatment groups. The live birth rates reported in this study were 34% and 40% for laparoscopic ovarian drilling and other medical treatment groups, respectively. The other treatment groups studied were clomiphene citrate and tamoxifen, gonadotropins, and aromatase inhibitors. Benefits of the procedure include no increased risk of multifetal gestation or ovarian hyperstimulation. Limitations of the procedure include the lack of impact on metabolic profile as well as common surgical related risks, such as postoperative adhesion formation or potential decreased ovarian reserve.

OBSTETRIC EFFECTS

Pregnancy complications in women with PCOS include a higher incidence of gestational diabetes mellitus (40%–50%), gestational hypertensive disorders (5%), and infants who are small for gestational age (10%–15%).[38] The basis for these complications stems from obesity, altered glucose metabolism, and disturbances in uterine blood flow. Independent risk factors for obesity include spontaneous miscarriage, preeclampsia, gestational diets, congenital anomalies, fetal macrosomnia, cesarean delivery, and wound complications after cesarean delivery. In one meta-analysis, women with PCOS when compared with controls showed a statistically significant higher risk of developing gestational diabetes mellitus, preeclampsia, and preterm birth. These risks were found to be independent of weight and age. Prevention strategies include pregestational weight loss and optimal glycemic control in those women with glucose intolerance or diabetes. Intrapregnancy weight gain should be closely supervised. The Institute of Medicine established specific guidelines for weight gain in pregnancy depending on BMI. Individuals of normal weight should gain between 11.3 and 13.6 kg (25 and 30 lb), whereas overweight individuals should gain between 6.8 and 11.3 kg (15 and 25 lb). Obese females should gain no more than 6.8 kg (15 lb).[39] Several studies have examined the role of bariatric surgery in the pregestational period. Bariatric surgery may alleviate the obstetric risks of these women. However, the general recommendation for those women who have undergone bariatric surgery is to wait 12 to 18 months after surgery before conceiving.[1] During this period, individuals experience the greatest amount of rapid weight loss, and there is concern regarding malabsorption of micronutrients, which may result in poor fetal growth.

It was previously believed that women with PCOS were at increased risk of spontaneous abortion. However, spontaneous abortion rates in PCOS women are comparable with those in other subfertile populations. The rate has been found to correlate more with the incidence of obesity in this group. PPCOS I quoted rates of spontaneous miscarriage ranging from 8% to 21%, which is consistent with rates of other subfertile women.[1] In PPCOS II, in which the mean BMI was 35, the spontaneous miscarriage rate was about 28% in both arms of the study.[23]

SUMMARY

PCOS is a multifaceted disease, which commonly affects fertility. Management strategies for overweight and obese women with PCOS who desire fertility should include weight loss. Even a small reduction in body weight can improve ovulatory function and pregnancy rate and reduce adverse obstetric outcomes. New data suggest that letrozole should be considered as the new first-line medical treatment of anovulatory infertility in PCOS over clomiphene citrate. Second-line treatments for anovulatory infertility include IVF, gonadotropins, or ovarian drilling. Metformin is no longer recommended as monotherapy or in adjunct to clomiphene for ovulation induction, because it has not been shown to improve live birth rates. Limiting factors of all these treatments must always be considered and may include OHSS, multifetal gestation, and medication-specific side effects.

REFERENCES

1. Rotterdam ESHRE/ASRM-Sponsored PCOS Consensus Workshop Group. Revised 2003 consensus on diagnostic criteria and long-term health risks related to polycystic ovary syndrome (PCOS). Hum Reprod 2004;19:41–7.
2. Polycystic Ovary Syndrome. ACOG Practice Bulletin. Number 108. American College of Obstetricians and Gynecologists, October 2009. Reaffirmed 2013.
3. Legro R, Arslanian S, Ehrmann D, et al. Diagnosis and treatment of polycystic ovary syndrome: an Endocrine Society clinical practice guideline. J Clin Endocrinol Metab 2013;98:4565–92.
4. Laven JS, Imani B, Eijkemans MJ, et al. New approach to polycystic ovary syndrome and other forms of anovulatory infertility. Obstet Gynecol Surv 2002;57: 755–67.
5. Apter D. Endocrine and metabolic abnormalities in adolescents with a PCOS-like condition: consequences for adult reproduction. Trends Endocrinol Metab 1998; 9:58–61.
6. Chittenden BG, Fullerton G, Maheshwari A, et al. Polycystic ovary syndrome and the risk of gynaecological cancer: a systematic review. Reprod Biomed Online 2009;19:398–405.
7. Management of abnormal uterine bleeding associated with Ovulatory Dysfunction. ACOG Practice Bulletin, Number 136. American College of Obstetricians and Gynecologists, July 2013.
8. Jamal M, Gunay Y, Capper A. Roux-en-Y gastric bypass ameliorates polycystic ovary syndrome and dramatically improves conception rates: a 9-year analysis. Surg Obes Relat Dis 2012;8:440–4.
9. Ghandi S, Aflatoonian A, Tabibneiad N, et al. The effects of metformin or orlistat on obese women with polycystic ovary syndrome: a prospective randomized open-label study. J Assist Reprod Genet 2011;28:591–6.
10. Zimmerman Y, Zijkemans M, Coelingh B. The effect of oral contraceptives on testosterone levels in healthy women: a systematic review and meta-analysis. Hum Reprod Update 2014;20:40–62.
11. Tang T, Norman R, Balen A, et al. Insulin-sensitizing drugs (metformin, troglitazone, rosiglitazone, pioglitazone, D-chiro-inositol) for polycystic ovary syndrome. Cochrane Database Syst Rev 2003;2:CD003053.
12. Raval A, Hunter T, Stuckey B, et al. Statins for women with polycystic ovary syndrome not actively trying to conceive. Cochrane Database Syst Rev 2011;(10):CD008565.
13. Sirmans S, Pate K. Epidemiology, diagnosis and management of polycystic ovary syndrome. Clin Epidemiol 2014;6:1–13.

14. Hatch R. Hirsutism: implications, etiology and management. Am J Obstet Gynecol 1981;140:815–30.
15. Dinh Q, Sinclair R. Female pattern hair loss: current treatment concepts. Clin Interv Aging 2007;2:189–99.
16. Balfour J, McClellan K. Topical eflornithine. Am J Clin Dermatol 2001;2:197–201.
17. Thiboutot D, Chen W. Update and future of hormonal therapy in acne. Dermatology 2003;206:870–2.
18. Azziz R. The time has come to simplify the evaluation of the hirsute patient. Fertil Steril 2000;74:870–2.
19. Tobechi E, Arch E, Berson D. Hormonal treatment of acne in women. J Clin Aesthet Dermatol 2009;2:16–22.
20. Essan P, Wickham E, Nuney J. Dermatology of androgen-related disorders. Clin Dermatol 2006;24:289–98.
21. Futterweit W, Dunaif A, Yen H. The prevalence of hyperandrogenism in 109 consecutive female patients with diffuse alopecia. J Am Acad Dermatol 1988; 19:831–6.
22. Kaufman K. Androgen metabolism affects hair growth in androgenic alopecia. Dermatol Clin 1996;14:697–711.
23. Legro R, Brzyski R, Diamond M, et al. Letrozole versus clomiphene for infertility in the polycystic ovary syndrome. N Engl J Med 2014;371:119–29.
24. Huber-Buchholz M, Carey D, Norman R. Restoration of reproductive potential by lifestyle modification in obese polycystic ovarian syndrome: role of insulin sensitivity and luteinizing hormone. J Clin Endocrinol Metab 1999;84:1470–4.
25. Moran L, Hutchinson S, Normal R. Lifestyle changes in women with polycystic ovary syndrome. Cochrane Database Syst Rev 2011;(7):CD007506.
26. Legro R, Kunselman A, Brzyski R, et al. The Pregnancy in Polycystic Ovary Syndrome II (PPCOS II) trial: rationale and design of a double-blind randomized trial of clomiphene citrate and letrozole for the treatment of infertility in women with polycystic ovary syndrome. Contemp Clin Trials 2012;33:470–81.
27. Hurst B, Hickman J, Matthews M, et al. Novel clomiphene "stair-step" protocol reduces time to ovulation in women with polycystic ovarian syndrome. Am J Obstet Gynecol 2009;200:510.
28. Deveci C, Demir B, Sengul O, et al. Clomiphene citrate 'stair-step' protocol vs. traditional protocol in patients with polycystic ovary syndrome: a randomized controlled trial. Arch Gynecol Obstet 2014. [Epub ahead of print].
29. Guzick D. Ovulation induction management of PCOS. Clin Obstet Gynecol 2007; 50:255–67.
30. Diamond M, Kruger M, Santoro N, et al. Endometrial shedding effect on conception and live birth in women with polycystic ovary syndrome. Obstet Gynecol 2012;119:902–8.
31. Engmann L, Diluigi A, Schmidt D, et al. The use of gonadotropin-releasing hormone (GnRH) agonist to induce oocyte maturation after cotreatment with GnRH antagonist in high-risk patients undergoing in vitro fertilization prevents the risk of ovarian hyperstimulation syndrome: a prospective randomized controlled study. Fertil Steril 2008;89:84–91.
32. Palomba S, Falbo A, La Sala G. Metformin and gonadotropins for ovulation induction in patients with polycystic ovary syndrome: a systematic review with meta-analysis of randomized controlled trials. Reprod Biol Endocrinol 2014;12:3.
33. The Thessaloniki ESHRE/ASRM- Sponsored PCOS Consensus Workshop Group. Consensus on infertility treatment related to polycystic ovary syndrome. Hum Reprod 2007;23:462–77.

34. Kuivasaari-Pirinen P, Hippeläinen M, Hakkarainen H, et al. Cumulative baby take-home rate among women with PCOS treated by IVF. Gynecol Endocrinol 2010;26: 582–9.
35. Bailey A, Hawkins LK, Missmer S, et al. Effect of body mass index on in vitro fertilization outcomes in women with polycystic ovary syndrome. Am J Obstet Gynecol 2014;211:163.
36. Palomba S, Falbo A, La Sala G. Effects of metformin in women with polycystic ovary syndrome treated with gonadotropins for in vitro fertilization and intracytoplasmic sperm injection cycles: a systematic review and meta-analysis of randomized controlled trials. BJOG 2013;120:267–76.
37. Farquhar C, Brown J, Marjoribanks J. Laparoscopic drilling by diathermy or laser for ovulation induction in anovulatory polycystic ovary syndrome. Cochrane Database Syst Rev 2012;(6):CD001122.
38. Qin J, Pang L, Li M, et al. Obstetric complications in women with polycystic ovary syndrome: a systematic review and meta-analysis. Reprod Biol Endocrinol 2013; 26:11–56.
39. Leddy M, Power ML, Schulkin J. The impact of maternal obesity on maternal and fetal health. Rev Obstet Gynecol 2008;1:170–8.

Clinical Management of Leiomyoma

Carter Owen, MD[a], Alicia Y. Armstrong, MD, MHSCR[b],*

KEYWORDS

- Fibroids • Leiomyoma • Pathophysiology • Clinical management • Research

KEY POINTS

- Uterine leiomyoma, benign monoclonal tumors, afflict an estimated 60% of reproductive-aged women, with higher rates among African American women.
- Leiomyomas are associated with significant medical costs, impaired fertility potential, obstetric complications, and gynecologic morbidity.
- Currently, the effective clinical management of leiomyoma is limited by the fact that hysterectomy is the only cure.
- New methods of diagnosis, medical and surgical treatments, as well as interventional radiology and treatment methods are being examined.

INTRODUCTION

In this section, the demographic characteristics and costs of leiomyoma are examined to provide the reader with a brief review of the scope of the problem.

Uterine leiomyomas are exceedingly common, with 60% of reproductive-aged women being affected, and 80% of women developing disease during their lifetime.[1] More than 600,000 hysterectomies are performed annually, and fibroids are the leading indication for hysterectomy in the United States.[2] The annual costs associated with fibroids are estimated at 4 to 10 billion dollars. Estimated lost work-hour costs ranged from $1.55 to 17.2 billion annually. Obstetric outcomes that were attributed to fibroid tumors resulted in a cost of $238 million to $7.76 billion each year.[3]

In addition to the gynecologic complications associated with leiomyoma, fibroids are associated with 10% of cases of infertility. In a little less than 5% of patients, leiomyomas are the only cause of infertility.[4] Among women undergoing assisted

The authors have nothing to disclose.
[a] Program in Reproductive and Adult Endocrinology, Eunice Kennedy Shriver National Institute of Child Health and Human Development, National Institutes of Health, Building 10, CRC, Bethesda, MD 20892, USA; [b] Contraception Discovery and Development Branch, Eunice Kennedy Shriver National Institute of Child Health and Human Development, National Institutes of Health, 6100 Executive Boulevard, Rockville, MD 20852, USA
* Corresponding author. Room 8B13J, 6100 Executive Boulevard, Rockville, MD 20852.
E-mail address: armstroa@mail.nih.gov

Obstet Gynecol Clin N Am 42 (2015) 67–85
http://dx.doi.org/10.1016/j.ogc.2014.09.009
0889-8545/15/$ – see front matter Published by Elsevier Inc.
obgyn.theclinics.com

reproductive technologies, there is clinical evidence to support an association of cavity distortion by submucosal and intramural leiomyoma and of decreased implantation rates after embryo transfer. The clinical data have been considered compelling enough to support a recommendation of myomectomy before IVF.[5] Recent leiomyoma investigations have elucidated previously unknown demographic factors. The age of onset of disease, for example, has been demonstrated to occur at a younger age based on ultrasound evaluations in asymptomatic women. In a recent study of African American and Caucasian women less than 30 years of age, the overall prevalence of leiomyoma based on transvaginal ultrasound was 14.9%. Leiomyomas were more common among African American women than Caucasian women (25.6% vs 6.9%).[6] These findings challenge the traditional dogma that fibroids are uncommon in women under the age of 30.

Age at menarche has also been shown to be an important demographic characteristic that can help identify women at risk for the development of leiomyoma. In a large epidemiologic study of 5023 women screened by ultrasound, early age at first menses had a positive association with fibroid size, type, and location, with a stronger association noted for multiple fibroids.[7] These findings are consistent with earlier studies that identified early age at menarche as a risk factor for the development of leiomyomas.[8]

Obesity has been shown to be a risk factor for fibroid development and may partially explain the increased incidence of leiomyoma among groups that have a high rate of obesity. In a retrospective cohort study, 50% of women with fibroids were found to be obese and 16% were morbidly obese compared with a 25% rate of obesity and a 7.2% rate of morbid obesity in the general population.[9] In a more recent publication, the risk of uterine fibroid development was reported to be 3 times greater for women who weigh more than 70 kg, compared with women who weigh less than 50 kg.[10] Given the increasing incidence of obesity in the United States, an associated increase in the incidence of leiomyoma can be anticipated.

Like pregnancy, family history has been a subject of debate. A recent study suggested that self-reported family history may not be a reliable marker for a high risk of leiomyoma development. In a study of 1072 women (660 African American, 412 Caucasian), self-reported family history of fibroids was not found to be a useful tool for identifying high-risk women.[11]

In summary, some of the most common demographic risk factors include African American race, obesity, and age at menarche. Other factors, such as parity and family history, remain a subject of debate. Additional epidemiologic factors, such as diet, particularly vitamin D deficiency, and environmental toxins, are the subject of ongoing investigations. Further research is needed to identify additional demographic characteristics that are associated with fibroid development. This information will be helpful in counseling patients about their risk of disease. As effective prophylactic treatments are developed, prospective intervention may be possible.

PATHOPHYSIOLOGY

In this section, the pathophysiology of leiomyoma, including molecular mechanisms and genetics, is discussed. In examining the gross appearance of leiomyoma as well as the molecular structure, it has become clear that these benign tumors are composed of altered collagen fibrils, resulting in an altered extracellular matrix (ECM) compared with adjacent myometrium. The distorted ECM is thought to contribute to the increased rigidity of leiomyoma compared with normal myometrium. This understanding of the ECM in the context of a dynamic uterine muscle has led to the theory that molecular forces likely play a role in the development and growth of leiomyoma.[12]

It is well known that sex steroids, estrogen and progesterone, promote the growth of uterine fibroids.[13] However, Peddada and colleagues[14] have reported that leiomyomas grow and shrink at different rates within the same woman despite the similar exposure to hormonal milieu. Actually, twice as much variation was noted within women as between women highlighting the multifactorial mechanisms involved in leiomyoma progression.

The observation that leiomyomas resemble scar tissue in conjunction with the discovery that numerous cytokines and integrins are altered in leiomyoma compared with adjacent myometrium has highlighted the likely importance of tissue remodeling, fibrosis, and the inflammatory response in the development and progression of these tumors. It may be that the disordered ECM of leiomyoma arises in the uterus as an altered response to noxious stimuli. In recent years, investigators have also elucidated that leiomyomas exist in a state of severe hypoxia compared with normal myometrium. The hypoxia is thought to result in part from abnormal angiogenesis and resulting vasculature, which also could be part of an overarching altered inflammatory response.[15,16] Still another theory put forward by Cramer and colleagues is that a precursor lesion in the myometrium may lead to the development of uterine leiomyoma. Cramer and colleagues[17] found an association between seedling leiomyoma (<1 cm) and myometrial hyperplasia.

Cytogenetic studies have advanced the understanding of the possible causes of leiomyoma. It is known that leiomyomas are monoclonal in origin and that approximately 40% to 50% harbor a cytogenetic abnormality. Most abnormalities have been found in chromosomes 6, 7, 12, and 14.[18]

The initial cytogenetic studies used analysis of the X-linked glucose-6-phosphate dehydrogenase isoenzyme to demonstrate that multiple leiomyomas within a single uterus harbor random patterns of X-inactivation, suggesting that each tumor develops independently.[19] In approximately 20% of karyotypically abnormal leiomyomas, a t(12;14) chromosomal translocation is seen.[20] Other mesenchymal solid tumors (eg, breast fibroadenomas and lipomas) exhibit translocations involving the same region of Chromosome 12, supporting the hypothesis that the gene mapped to this area is important for tumor development.[21] HMGA2, a member of the high mobility gene group linked to self-renewal ability, has been mapped to this area and is found to be overexpressed in uterine leiomyoma.[22] Similarly, rearrangements in chromosome 6p21, occurring in less than 5% of leiomyoma, have been found to lead to upregulation of another member of the high mobility gene group, HGMA1.[23]

Aside from the known chromosomal abnormalities listed above, a variety of other less frequent cytogenetic abnormalities have been identified in leiomyoma.[18] A recent investigation of the genetics of leiomyoma as it relates to leiomyoma as a health disparity issue found that many genes were differentially expressed in the leiomyoma of older black compared with older white women.[24] One interesting finding of the study was that CAIII, a gene encoding an enzyme that serves to buffer cellular acid-base, was the most highly expressed gene in the leiomyoma of black women compared with leiomyoma from white women. These results could explain how the aberrant smooth muscle cells of leiomyoma survive in such a hypoxic and acidic environment and develop such a severe phenotype in black women.[24]

The existence of a disparity of leiomyoma phenotypes between black and white women underlines a likely genetic liability of the disease in certain groups that cannot be explained by variations in demographics alone. In addition, an inherited factor for certain types of leiomyoma is certain with the germline mutation having been identified such as patients with hereditary leiomyomatosis and renal cell carcinoma. However, the marked prevalence of leiomyoma overall suggests that genetics is only one component of the overall cause of leiomyoma and further investigation is still needed in this area.

DIAGNOSIS AND ASSESSMENT

In this section, the diagnosis and assessment of leiomyoma, including clinical symptoms and the role of imaging, are discussed.

Most women with uterine fibroids are asymptomatic[25,26]; however, women can experience abnormal uterine bleeding (AUB), pelvic pain, bulk symptoms, reproductive dysfunction, sexual dysfunction, and urologic complications. It has been estimated that approximately 20% to 50% of patients with uterine leiomyoma experience symptoms credited to the presence of myomas.[27,28] It is well known that the symptoms caused by uterine fibroids significantly impact women's quality of life and well-being.[29] With so many women affected by leiomyoma, this condition accounts for a significant burden of disease. Most women are diagnosed with leiomyoma after they present for the evaluation of symptoms, during infertility work-up, or incidentally at the time of other diagnostic imaging.[30,31] It has been estimated in one study that each year approximately 1% of reproductive-aged women affected by uterine leiomyoma will present for consultation with a provider because of their bothersome symptoms.[32]

The most common symptom of leiomyoma, occurring in 30% of women with the disease, is AUB. Excessive bleeding can have a significant impact on quality of life because it may interfere with one's personal and work life and be the precipitating factor in the development of other medical issues, such as iron deficiency anemia.[33] In some cases, AUB from uterine leiomyoma can lead to acute, life-threatening hemorrhage requiring emergent blood transfusion and hospitalization. The cause of AUB in the presence of leiomyoma is poorly understood, but many groups have proposed various theories including obstruction from fibroids leading to venule ectasia in the endometrium,[34] increased surface area of the endometrium,[35] and the dysregulation of local growth factors and aberrant angiogenesis within the uterus and endometrium.[36]

In addition, women with uterine leiomyoma may present with symptoms of pelvic pain, dysmenorrhea, and dyspareunia. One population-based cross-sectional study looking at women who were not seeking care found that women with ultrasound-confirmed fibroids were more likely to report moderate to severe dyspareunia and noncyclic pelvic pain. Interestingly, women without fibroids were just as likely as women with fibroids to report moderate or severe dysmenorrhea. This study also showed that there was no association between the number and total volume of fibroids and pelvic pain.[37]

The suspected diagnosis of leiomyoma may be based in some cases on the palpation of an enlarged irregular uterine contour on pelvic examination in the office.[38] Women may experience urinary frequency, difficulty emptying the bladder, or, in rare cases, hydronephrosis and chronic kidney disease.[39] With posterior pressure from bulky leiomyoma, the patient may suffer from low back pain or constipation.[40] It is important to take a careful history during the assessment of uterine fibroids, because the severity of symptoms will often inform the management of leiomyoma.

Uterine leiomyomas in some women who were previously undiagnosed are discovered during infertility evaluation. Uterine fibroids may be found in approximately 5% to

10% of infertile women. However, when all other factors are excluded, it is estimated that only 2% to 3% of infertility is attributed to uterine fibroids.[25,41] Systematic reviews have shown that submucosal and intracavitary fibroids are associated with decreased clinical pregnancy and implantation rates and that removal appears to improve fertility.[42,43] Consensus is that the proximity of uterine fibroids to the uterine cavity determines detrimental effects on infertility, but there is still much work to be done to elucidate the impact of intramural fibroids on fertility.

Once leiomyoma is suspected by history, physical examination, or incidental discovery, imaging should be undertaken to confirm the presence, location, characterization, and size of uterine leiomyoma. This process is often called uterine mapping or leiomyoma mapping. Although uterine fibroids may be detected on computed tomographic scans or at the time of hysterosalpingogram, there is little to no role for either of these studies in the evaluation of leiomyoma. Ultrasound, both transvaginal and transabdominal, is most frequently used in the assessment of leiomyoma because of its low cost and accessibility.[44] Transvaginal ultrasonography alone has been shown to have sensitivity for detecting uterine fibroids in the range of 65% to 99%.[45–47] There is improved sensitivity of detecting submucosal myomas with the addition of sonohysterography.[48] However, one the major limitations of ultrasonography, as demonstrated above in the wide range of sensitivity, is its operator-dependence, resulting in poor reproducibility as compared with MRI.[49–52] In addition, subserosal fibroids as well as small fibroids may not be identified by transvaginal ultrasound.[53]

MRI is a more costly modality, but is thought to be more exact in its capacity for leiomyoma mapping, especially in large uteri (>375 mL) and in uteri with greater than 4 myomas.[47] MRI is also better able to distinguish uterine leiomyoma from leiomyosarcoma and adenomyosis.[54–56] In addition, because of the precise resolution and anatomic detail afforded by MRI, 69% of benign histologic subtypes of leiomyoma can be identified, including cellular, degenerated, and necrotizing leiomyoma as well as lipoleiomyoma and acutely infarcting leiomyoma.[57]

Proper diagnosis and assessment of uterine fibroids play an important role in deciding the management plans for patients.

FIBROIDS MEDICAL THERAPY

Currently, hysterectomy is the only cure for fibroids, which underscores the need for identification of effective nonsurgical medical treatments, with high efficacy, and a desirable side-effect profile. This section reviews the use of medical treatments, both as adjuvant therapy and as primary therapy. The discussion focuses on gonadotrophin-releasing hormone (GnRH) analogues, selective progesterone receptor (SPRM) modulators, and aromatase inhibitors (AI). The use of levonorgestrel-containing IUDs (LNG-IUS) is also reviewed.

Adjuvant Therapy

For women with anemia, or fibroids that are extremely large, or located in positions that will make surgical removal challenging, adjuvant preoperative medical therapy may be clinically helpful. GnRH analogues (eg, leuprolide) have been most extensively studied for this indication, and the discussion focuses on these agents. Studies of GnRH analogue effect have shown that fibroid tumor shrinkage is proportional to the number of estrogen receptor-positive cells, suggesting that GnRH analogues mediate their effect via reduction in estrogen levels.[58]

The most comprehensive review of the clinical utility of GnRH analogues is the Cochrane Systematic Review of the role of GnRH analogues before hysterectomy or myomectomy. This review showed a significant improvement in both preoperative and postoperative hemoglobin when GnRH analogues were used before surgery. Operative time for hysterectomy was reduced, and a greater number of patients undergoing hysterectomy were able to have a vaginal hysterectomy. Blood loss, the use of vertical skin incisions, and hospital stay duration were reduced for both myomectomy and hysterectomy.[59]

GnRH analogues are the only drugs that are Food and Drug Administration (FDA)-approved as medical fibroid therapeutics for the indication of preoperative adjunctive therapy to control bleeding, decrease fibroid size, and improve preoperative anemia. Despite FDA approval, the cost, the hypoestrogenic effects, rapid regrowth after cessation of medication, and bone demineralization after long-term use limit GnRH analogues to short-term adjuvant therapy in most patients.[60]

Multiple basic science and clinical investigations have provided evidence that progesterone and the progesterone receptor may play a role in enhancing proliferative activity in leiomyoma. This growing body of literature supports a potential therapeutic role for antiprogestins and drugs that modulate progesterone receptor activity, such as SPRMs.[61]

Much of the early clinical research with selective progesterone modulators involved the use of mifepristone and asoprisnil. Both drugs have been shown to be efficacious in reducing fibroid size and improving fibroid associated symptoms.[62] More recently, ulipristal acetate (UPA), approved for emergency contraception, has been the focus of clinical investigations. UPA has been shown to improve quality of life, reduce fibroid volume, and induce amenorrhea in most of the women treated and is now approved for clinical use in both Europe and Canada.[63,64] In a double-blind study comparing UPA to leuprolide acetate, UPA controlled bleeding in nearly 100% of women, and they became amenorrheic 2 weeks earlier than women treated with leuprolide. UPA was associated with reduction in fibroid volume of approximately 25% when compared with placebo. A major advantage of UPA over leuprolide is the lack of hypoestrogenic side effects and bone loss. These differences between UPA and leuprolide may make UPA a preferred choice for preoperative adjuvant therapy.[65]

The endometrial effects of SPRMs have been a major concern with the use of these agents. Theoretically, SPRM modulators may cause blockade of progesterone action on the endometrium, and inhibition of ovulation could result in unopposed estrogen. Although initial histologic findings associated with the drug were concerning for hyperplasia, more recent histologic assessments have demonstrated histologic changes that are unique to SPRMs, termed progesterone-associated endometrial changes, which appear to be benign in nature.[66] More recent studies have not shown atypical hyperplasia in patients receiving SPRMs, and progesterone-associated changes regress after cessation of therapy, but the long-term effect of these drugs on the endometrium has not been established.

AI represent a class of antiestrogens that block the synthesis of estrogen. AI have become standard adjuvant therapy for postmenopausal women with estrogen receptor–positive breast cancer, as a result of their ability to produce in situ estrogen inhibition as compared with the indirect inhibition induced by GnRH agonists.[67] These properties also made AI very attractive candidates for the medical treatment of leiomyoma.

Basic science studies in the mid-1990s revealed that aromatase mRNA was detected in more than 90% of fibroids, but was undetectable in myometrial tissues from normal uteri.[68] Other investigators found that there were racial differences, with leiomyoma tissue from African American women having the highest levels of aromatase expression. These differences may explain, in part, the differences in the higher prevalence and earlier incidence in African American women. It also suggests that African American women may be more responsive to aromatase inhibitor therapy.[69]

Multiple clinical studies have shown a reduction in fibroid size and improvement of symptoms with aromatase inhibitor therapy. In a small prospective clinical trial, Gurates and colleagues[70] found that letrozole significantly decreased fibroid size and relieved heavy menstrual bleeding without changing bone mineral density. Several other investigators found that anastrozole was effective in reducing fibroid volume and improving symptoms without changing follicle-stimulating hormone (FSH) or estradiol levels.[71] The unique properties of AI also make it a therapeutic option in postmenopausal women with leiomyoma. In a study of obese postmenopausal women with fibroids and persistent bleeding, Kaunitz[72] demonstrated that anastrozole reduced fibroid size and caused endometrial thinning and cessation of bleeding.

Although AI have great potential as a medical therapy for leiomyoma and have several advantages over GnRH analogues, a recent *Cochrane Review* concluded that evidence was insufficient to support the use of AI drugs in the treatment of women with uterine fibroids.[73] Additional clinical studies, with larger numbers of subjects, will be necessary to determine the long-term safety, optimal treatment regimens, and impact on reproductive function.

No randomized controlled trials of LNG-IUS in women with fibroids have been published; however, multiple clinical studies suggest that bleeding markedly decreases in women with leiomyoma that have heavy menstrual bleeding. In a systematic review by Zapata and colleagues,[74] they reported that menstrual blood loss decreased in the 11 studies included in their analysis. These investigations also demonstrated an increase in hemoglobin, hematocrit, and ferritin. Some, but not all, studies showed an increase in expulsion rates. In the 6 prospective noncomparative studies, expulsion rates varied from 0% to 20%. Unlike uterine bleeding, fibroid volumes measured by MRI were not decreased in women using LNG-IUS.[75] In women with a need for contraception who do not desire surgery, or who need to correct their anemia before surgery, the LNG-IUS is an option that should be offered to these patients.

UTERINE ARTERY EMBOLIZATION

Uterine artery embolization (UAE) is a widely accepted, nonsurgical technique used to treat symptomatic uterine fibroids. This technique has been endorsed by the American College of Obstetricians and Gynecologists as safe and effective for women with uterine fibroids who are appropriately selected.[76] UAE is ideal for women with symptomatic uterine fibroids who have medical management, are poor surgical candidates, wish to avoid surgery, or wish to retain their uterus.

Women seeking UAE most often complain of AUB, especially heavy menstrual bleeding, and bulk symptoms. In a randomized controlled trial that compared UAE to hysterectomy (EMMY trial), UAE was associated with a significantly shorter hospital stay and had a similar improvement in health-related quality of life compared with hysterectomy. However, women who underwent hysterectomy were significantly more satisfied with their received treatment.[77] Similar improvements in quality of life were seen in the REST trial, another multicenter randomized controlled trial performed in the United Kingdom comparing UAE with surgery (myomectomy or hysterectomy). The EMMY trial reported reintervention in the UAE group in 28% of patients and the REST trial reported a cumulative intervention rate of 32% with both trials following the patients for up to 5 years.[78] One analysis of trials examining UAE versus surgical intervention demonstrated that UAE is associated with a shorter hospital stay, a quicker return to activities, and a higher minor complication rate after discharge.[79]

Contraindications to UAE include on-going pregnancy and active uterine or adnexal infections. Allergy to intravenous contrast and renal insufficiency are relative contraindications and special considerations should be made for patients on anticoagulation medications. As with all therapies dealing with fibroids, physicians should consider size and location of myomas when counseling patients for UAE. Women with very large uteri (greater than 22-weeks size) may not have significant improvement in their symptoms after UAE, and cervical or broad ligament fibroids are less likely to respond to UAE because these fibroids are more likely to have collateral blood supplies.

According to the fibroid registry, the most common complication of UAE is severe pain requiring hospitalization. Postembolization syndrome, consisting of mild-to-moderate pain, low-grade fever, and malaise, is also very common following the procedure and is usually managed with analgesics and antipyretics. Sloughing of an embolized fibroid into the uterine cavity resulting in foul-smelling vaginal discharge will be experienced by 2.2% to 7% of patients.[80] Mortality resulting from UAE is exceedingly rare, with only a few cases ever reported. The most common potentially fatal complication is pulmonary embolism (1 in 400 patients). The potential detrimental effect of UAE on the ovaries is also an area of controversy. There is a 3% chance of amenorrhea in young women attributed to impairment of ovarian function from embolization of collateral blood supply.[81] This risk seems to be age-related and, in some women not desiring future childbearing, amenorrhea could be the therapeutic goal. The EMMY randomized clinical trial of UAE versus hysterectomy reported similar ovarian impairment as measured by preprocedure and postprocedure antimullerian hormone and FSH levels.[82]

The effects of UAE on fertility and pregnancy are still areas of controversy. At present, if fibroids are determined to be the cause of infertility, then myomectomy is the preferred treatment. One of the best studies to investigate the effects of UAE on fertility was a randomized trial in 121 women with fibroids desiring fertility undergoing myomectomy versus UAE and followed for up to 2 years. This study found that women were significantly more able to achieve pregnancy after myomectomy (78%) versus UAE (50%). They also found that UAE was associated with a greater risk of spontaneous abortion.[83] In addition, some authors have suggested a concern that UAE increases the complication rate during future pregnancies. One retrospective study examining pregnancies after UAE (n = 53) compared with myomectomy (n = 139) demonstrated that in the UAE group there was a higher rate of preterm birth, malpresentation, and cesarean section.[84] The Ontario multicenter trial included a cohort of 24 pregnancies occurring in women after UAE. They found a 12% risk of placentation complications (2 placenta previa and 1 placenta accreta) all occurring in nulliparous women with no other identified risk factors. Given the biologic plausibility of UAE leading to compromised endometrial perfusion and thus abnormal placentation, UAE should be recommended with caution for women desiring future fertility.[85]

In general, UAE is an excellent treatment option for women who have failed medical management, completed childbearing, have contraindications to surgery, or wish to avoid surgical intervention. More studies are needed to investigate the risks and benefits of UAE in women with infertility and those desiring future pregnancies. Based on the current evidence, UAE should be offered with caution and only after careful counseling to women desiring future fertility.

MAGNETIC RESONANCE–GUIDED FOCUSED ULTRASOUND SURGERY

In 2004, the FDA approved the first magnetic resonance–guided focused ultrasound surgery (MRgFUS) device as a noninvasive thermal ablation therapy for uterine fibroids. The technology uses MRI guidance to map and monitor high-intensity ultrasound-focused ablation of fibroid tumors. The goal of therapy is to achieve an increase in temperature within the fibroid leading to coagulation necrosis while avoiding patient discomfort and damage to surrounding structures (eg, bowel, bladder, neurovascular bundles).[86]

The ideal candidate for this therapy has symptomatic fibroids, which are usually limited to a few moderately sized fibroids (4–6 cm) or a single fibroid no more than 10 cm, has low signal intensity on T2-weighted MRI, and can be safely accessed by the ultrasound beam (no more than 12 cm from abdominal wall and no closer than 4 cm to sacrum). The patient must be able to lie prone for the therapy, which typically takes up to 3 hours, and receive intravenous conscious sedation, which is used to limit patient movement. Patients are typically excluded if they have serious health complications, have contraindications to MRI such as claustrophobia or implants, have significant abdominal scarring, have very large uteri (greater than 24-weeks size), or have pedunculated, nonenhancing, or heavily calcified fibroids.[87] In one study of women with large fibroids (>10 cm), treatment with GnRH agonist before MRgFUS improved treatment success by shrinking the fibroid to a more manageable size. GnRH agonists also decrease vascularity, which has been shown to increase the destructive effect of the thermal ablation.[88]

MRgFUS is usually well-tolerated with the recent studies showing no serious side effects and few minor complications, including abdominal pain, skin burns, and sciatic nerve paresthesia.[89] MRgFUS has been shown to improve quality of life and symptom severity scores, which most authors associate with the increased nonperfusion volume of the treated fibroids seen on MRI.[86] Initial FDA labeling of the MRgFUS device stated that it was for women who had completed child-bearing.[90] However, there have been 35 reported successful pregnancies without increased complications in women post-MRgFUS, which have raised the question of whether this technology, given its noninvasive approach, may actually be the treatment of choice for women who desire future fertility.[86] More studies are needed to address this question and determine the role for MRgFUS in the treatment of uterine fibroids.

SURGICAL THERAPIES

For women who desire surgery, the most important considerations are size and location (**Fig. 1**) of the fibroids and fertility potential. Although hysterectomy is the only cure, myomectomy is the only viable surgical option for women who want to maintain an option for future pregnancies. This section reviews surgical options, with a focus on patient selection and outcomes.

Patients who elect conservative surgery should be apprised of their risk of recurrence and likelihood of eventual hysterectomy. Although a precise individual risk cannot be identified, the literature suggests a recurrence rate of fibroids of nearly 60%, with most of the fibroids recurring between 3 and 5 years after surgery.[91] Women who are at risk for diminished ovarian reserve, or who have other infertility factors, should be offered assessment to help them in the decision to proceed with conservative surgery.

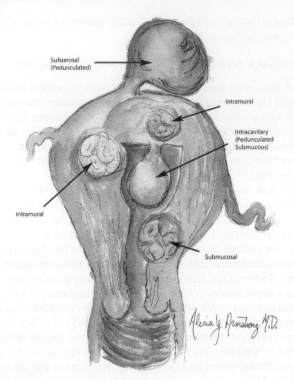

Subserosal
(Pedunculated)

Intramural

Intracavitary
(Pedunculated
Submucous)

Intramural

Submucosal

Alecia J. Armstrong, M.D.

Fig. 1. Locations of fibroid tumors.

Location of leiomyoma is a significant determinant of surgical route, and appropriate diagnostic imaging should be performed before selecting surgical approach (see **Fig. 1**). The best candidates for hysteroscopic myomectomy are patients with submucosal fibroids less than 3 cm, with greater than 50% of the fibroid being intracavitary. Type 0 (entirely intracavitary) and type 1 (greater than 50% intracavitary) may be candidates for this surgical approach. Patients with type 2, less than 50% intracavitary, are better candidates for abdominal surgery.[92] Although surgical experience and expertise are important factors, there are little published objective data related to this variable.

The selection of distension media is an important factor, particularly when prolonged surgical times are anticipated. Because myometrial integrity is breached in the performance of myomectomy, these procedures are at greater risk of systemic absorption. Carbon dioxide should only be used for diagnostic and not operative hysteroscopy. The maximum volumes for various types of distention media are shown in **Table 1**. Injection of dilute vasopressin solution preoperatively can decrease distending media absorption. Saline has the lowest risk of hyponatremia and hypo-osmolarity, but it requires the use of bipolar instruments (see **Table 1**).

LAPAROSCOPIC AND ROBOTIC MYOMECTOMY

For appropriate candidates, laparoscopic myomectomy offers the advantage of lower blood loss, more rapid return to normal activities, shorter hospital stays, and a more cosmetically acceptable scar. A large multicenter trial and other clinical investigations have reported uterine rupture after laparoscopic myomectomy, and it has been

Table 1
Maximum volumes for hysteroscopic distension media

Media Type	Maximum Volume	Comment
Saline	2500 mL	Isotonic media should be used whenever possible to reduce risk of hyponatremia. Requires use of bipolar instruments
Glycine (low viscosity)	1000 mL	Fluid overload with low viscosity media can result in hypotonic hyponatremia
Dextran (high viscosity)	500 mL	Volumes as low as 300 mL associated with adverse outcomes. Dextran 70 associated with anaphylaxis. Can caramelize on instruments
Sorbitol (low viscosity)	1000 mL	
Mannitol (low viscosity)	1000 mL	

Data from AAGL Practice Report: Practice Guidelines for the Management of Hysteroscopic Distending Media. J Minimally Invasive Gynecology 2013. Available at: http://www.aagl.org/wp-content/uploads/2013/03/aagl-Practice-Guidelines-for-the-Management-of-Hysteroscopic-Distending-Media.pdf. Accessed September 25, 2014.

recommended that women with fibroids greater than 5 cm multiple myomas and deep intramural myomas consider abdominal myomectomy.[93] Although there are many advantages to laparoscopic myomectomy, mastery of this procedure often requires considerable training.

The introduction of robotic assistance has helped to facilitate the surgeon's ability to perform myomectomy laparoscopically. There is also the additional advantage of expanding the number of patients who are candidates for laparoscopic myomectomy. Unfortunately, long-term outcomes data for alleviation of symptoms, residual fibroid burden, subsequent fertility, and patient satisfaction are lacking for robotic-assisted myomectomy.

ABDOMINAL MYOMECTOMY

Abdominal myomectomy is the preferred surgical option when hysteroscopy or laparoscopy is not an option, or the patient has another indication for laparotomy (**Fig. 2**). Other recommendations based on earlier studies suggested that women with more than 3 to 4 fibroids or total uterine size greater than 9 cm consider abdominal myomectomy. The increasing experience of surgeons and the advent of robotic technology have made it possible for women with larger uteri to avoid laparotomy. In a recent comparison of robotic surgery versus abdominal myomectomy, the uterine size limit was 20 weeks. Robotic surgery and abdominal myomectomy were equally efficacious in alleviating symptoms, but operative times were significantly longer with robotic surgery, and the residual fibroid burden was greater. Compared with abdominal myomectomy, patients undergoing robotic surgery had shorter hospital stays and a faster return to work.[93]

HYSTERECTOMY

For women who desire definitive therapy, there are several options, which include vaginal hysterectomy, total laparoscopic hysterectomy (TLH), laparoscopic-assisted vaginal hysterectomy (LAVH), and laparotomy. Like myomectomy, the surgical route is determined by size and location of the fibroids, surgeon experience, and patient

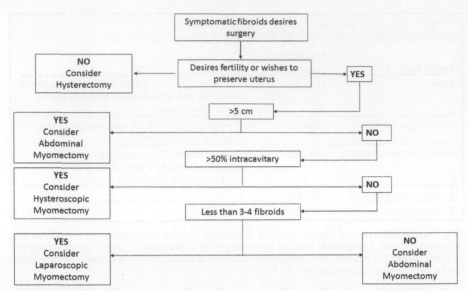

Fig. 2. Algorithm for surgical management of symptomatic fibroids. (*From* Heitmann RJ, Duke CM, Catherino WH, et al. Surgical treatments and outcomes. In: Segars JH, editor. Gynecology in practice: fibroids. Hoboken (NJ): Wiley-Blackwell, and imprint of John Wiley & Sons; 2013. p. 110; with permission.)

preference. In a recent randomized comparison of vaginal hysterectomy in Europe, TLH and LAVH for leiomyoma, the study found vaginal hysterectomy was the faster operative technique with lower blood loss and shorter time to discharge. The authors recommended that vaginal hysterectomy be considered the preferred approach. When vaginal hysterectomy is not feasible or salpingo-oophrectomy is required, LAVH or TLH should be considered.[94]

Morcellation allows appropriately selected patients to undergo minimally invasive surgery instead of laparotomy. Recent reports of dissemination of malignant tissue with this procedure, however, caused safety concerns. On April 17, 2014, the FDA issued a Safety Communication that discouraged the use of laparoscopic power morcellation in hysterectomy and myomectomy for fibroids. In May of 2014, American College of Obstetricians and Gynecologists released a Special Report stating that power morcellation remains an option for some women, but informed consent is critical.[95] The Special Report included the following:

- Minimally invasive surgery, including gynecologic power morcellation, continues to be an option for some patients undergoing hysterectomy or myomectomy;
- In women with strongly suspected or known uterine cancer, power morcellation should not be used;
- Preoperative evaluation and diagnosis play an important role when power morcellation is being considered; and
- Patient counseling and the informed consent process also play an important role. Physicians and patients considering power morcellation as an option during gynecologic surgery should discuss the risks, benefits, and alternatives.

The Special Report also called for further research, adequate training, development of safer methods, and a national prospective gynecologic power morcellation surgery registry to help acquire consistent and reliable data.

OUTCOMES

Rates of mortality for fibroid surgery are low, and the risk of serious complications is small. Surgical site infection rates vary from 1% to 11%, but most of these are superficial infections. Although rates of deep vein thromboses are high among surgical patients who do not receive prophylaxis, the risk of fatal pulmonary embolism is less than 1%. The risk of postoperative bleeding that requires transfusion is 2% after abdominal hysterectomy, but transfusion rates vary from 2% to 28% with myomectomy. Ninety-nine percent of women undergoing hysterectomy indicated that surgery improved or resolved their symptoms.

In conclusion, the specific indications for each surgical approach are subjective. Surgical route depends on the surgeon's experience, coexisting medical conditions, uterine size and location of the fibroids, and patient preference.

SUMMARY

Although hysterectomy remains the only cure for fibroids, there are several exciting candidates for medical therapies in the treatment of fibroids. Vitamin D, epigallocatechin gallate (EGCG), or green tea extract, compounds that increase retinoic acid and dietary supplements such as curcumin, all appear to have potential as nonsurgical therapies.

There is evidence to suggest that vitamin D inhibits growth, induces apoptosis in human leiomyoma cell cultures, and may act as an antifibrotic factor. Human studies examining vitamin D levels in healthy controls, and women with fibroids, indicate that there is a correlation with disease severity and vitamin D levels in women with symptomatic leiomyomas. There was a strong dose-response correlation, with women with more severe disease having lower levels of vitamin D.[96] These agents may have promise as a novel treatment option, or preventative therapy.

EGCG, or green tea extract, has been shown to inhibit proliferation of leiomyoma cells in vitro and in nude mice. EGCG has also been found to induce apoptosis as well as to inhibit cell proliferation through multiple signal transduction pathways, making it a potential medical therapy with a low side-effect profile.[97]

Another nutrition supplement that may have therapeutic benefit is curcumin, a dietary spice with antineoplastic activity. Curcumin inhibited leiomyoma cellular proliferation and decreased ECM proteoglycan expression in fibroids.[98] Distortions in the ECM are thought to contribute to the increased rigidity of leiomyoma compared with normal myometrium. This understanding of the ECM has led to the theory that molecular forces likely play a role in the development and growth of leiomyoma.[12] Given the ability of curcumin to decrease ECM proteoglycan expression, curcumin may be a potential medical therapy with very few safety issues.

Retinoids appear to modulate proliferative and apoptotic pathways in leiomyoma.[99] Abnormal ECM production appears to be linked to decreased endogenous retinoic acid, suggesting a possible role for compounds that increase endogenous retinoic acid. One such compound, liarozole, a retinoic acid metabolism blocking agent, may inhibit ECM formation through the retinoic pathway.

As the understanding of cellular differentiation pathways increases, new potential preventative and treatment modalities will be identified. For women who desire a surgical option, minimally invasive surgery technologies will offer options such as robotic and laparoscopic techniques, which have shorter hospital stays, lower complication rates, and shorter recovery times. Additional review and evaluation will be necessary to determine if some procedures, such as morcellation, offer more risk than benefit. Clinical research trial networks will facilitate the conduct of large clinical trials, which help to answer important questions about the potential benefit of new and existing clinical therapies.

REFERENCES

1. Baird DD, Dunson DB, Hill MC, et al. High cumulative incidence of uterine leiomyoma in black and white women: ultrasound evidence. Am J Obstet Gynecol 2003;188:100–7.
2. Moorman PG, Leppert P, Myers ER, et al. Comparison of characteristics of fibroids in African American and white women undergoing premenopausal hysterectomy. Fertil Steril 2013;99:768–76.e1.
3. Cardozo ER, Clark AD, Banks NK, et al. The estimated annual cost of uterine leiomyomata in the United States. Am J Obstet Gynecol 2012;206:211.e1–9.
4. Kolankaya A, Arici A. Myomas and assisted reproductive technologies: when and how to act? Obstet Gynecol Clin North Am 2006;33:145–52.
5. Sunkara SK, Khairy M, El-Toukhy T, et al. The effect of intramural fibroids without uterine cavity involvement on the outcome of IVF treatment: a systematic review and meta-analysis. Hum Reprod 2010;25:418–29.
6. Marsh EE, Ekpo GE, Cardozo ER, et al. Racial differences in fibroid prevalence and ultrasound findings in asymptomatic young women (18-30 years old): a pilot study. Fertil Steril 2013;99:1951–7.
7. Velez Edwards DR, Baird DD, Hartmann KE. Association of age at menarche with increasing number of fibroids in a cohort of women who underwent standardized ultrasound assessment. Am J Epidemiol 2013;178:426–33.
8. Dragomir AD, Schroeder JC, Connolly A, et al. Potential risk factors associated with subtypes of uterine leiomyomata. Reprod Sci 2010;17:1029–35.
9. Shikora SA, Niloff JM, Bistrian BR, et al. Relationship between obesity and uterine leiomyomata. Nutrition 1991;7:251–5.
10. Eltoukhi HM, Modi MN, Weston M, et al. The health disparities of uterine fibroid tumors for African American women: a public health issue. Am J Obstet Gynecol 2014;210:194–9.
11. Saldana TM, Moshesh M, Baird DD. Self-reported family history of leiomyoma: not a reliable marker of high risk. Ann Epidemiol 2013;23:286–90.
12. Norian JM, Owen CM, Taboas J, et al. Characterization of tissue biomechanics and mechanical signaling in uterine leiomyoma. Matrix Biol 2012;31:57–65.
13. Fields KR, Neinstein LS. Uterine myomas in adolescents: case reports and a review of the literature. J Pediatr Adolesc Gynecol 1996;9:195–8.
14. Peddada SD, Laughlin SK, Miner K, et al. Growth of uterine leiomyomata among premenopausal black and white women. Proc Natl Acad Sci U S A 2008;105: 19887–92.
15. Tal R, Segars JH. The role of angiogenic factors in fibroid pathogenesis: potential implications for future therapy. Hum Reprod Update 2014;20:194–216.
16. Mayer A, Hockel M, Wree A, et al. Lack of hypoxic response in uterine leiomyomas despite severe tissue hypoxia. Cancer Res 2008;68:4719–26.
17. Cramer SF, Mann L, Calianese E, et al. Association of seedling myomas with myometrial hyperplasia. Hum Pathol 2009;40:218–25.
18. Ligon AH, Morton CC. Leiomyomata: heritability and cytogenetic studies. Hum Reprod Update 2001;7:8–14.
19. Hashimoto K, Azuma C, Kamiura S, et al. Clonal determination of uterine leiomyomas by analyzing differential inactivation of the X-chromosome-linked phosphoglycerokinase gene. Gynecol Obstet Invest 1995;40:204–8.

20. Meloni AM, Surti U, Contento AM, et al. Uterine leiomyomas: cytogenetic and histologic profile. Obstet Gynecol 1992;80:209–17.
21. Calabrese G, Di Virgilio C, Cianchetti E, et al. Chromosome abnormalities in breast fibroadenomas. Genes Chromosomes Cancer 1991;3:202–4.
22. Schoenmakers EF, Wanschura S, Mols R, et al. Recurrent rearrangements in the high mobility group protein gene, HMGI-C, in benign mesenchymal tumours. Nat Genet 1995;10:436–44.
23. Tallini G, Vanni R, Manfioletti G, et al. HMGI-C and HMGI(Y) immunoreactivity correlates with cytogenetic abnormalities in lipomas, pulmonary chondroid hamartomas, endometrial polyps, and uterine leiomyomas and is compatible with rearrangement of the HMGI-C and HMGI(Y) genes. Lab Invest 2000;80:359–69.
24. Davis BJ, Risinger JI, Chandramouli GV, et al. Gene expression in uterine leiomyoma from tumors likely to be growing (from black women over 35) and tumors likely to be non-growing (from white women over 35). PLoS One 2013;8:e63909.
25. Buttram VC Jr, Reiter RC. Uterine leiomyomata: etiology, symptomatology, and management. Fertil Steril 1981;36:433–45.
26. Cramer SF, Patel A. The frequency of uterine leiomyomas. Am J Clin Pathol 1990;94:435–8.
27. Gupta S, Jose J, Manyonda I. Clinical presentation of fibroids. Best Pract Res Clin Obstet Gynaecol 2008;22:615–26.
28. Marino JL, Eskenazi B, Warner M, et al. Uterine leiomyoma and menstrual cycle characteristics in a population-based cohort study. Hum Reprod 2004;19:2350–5.
29. Spies JB, Coyne K, Guaou NG, et al. The UFS-QOL, a new disease-specific symptom and health-related quality of life questionnaire for leiomyomata. Obstet Gynecol 2002;99:290–300.
30. Levy G, Hill MJ, Beall S, et al. Leiomyoma: genetics, assisted reproduction, pregnancy and therapeutic advances. J Assist Reprod Genet 2012;29:703–12.
31. Levy G, Hill MJ, Plowden TC, et al. Biomarkers in uterine leiomyoma. Fertil Steril 2013;99:1146–52.
32. Marshall LM, Spiegelman D, Manson JE, et al. Risk of uterine leiomyomata among premenopausal women in relation to body size and cigarette smoking. Epidemiology 1998;9:511–7.
33. Wegienka G, Baird DD, Hertz-Picciotto I, et al. Self-reported heavy bleeding associated with uterine leiomyomata. Obstet Gynecol 2003;101:431–7.
34. Farrer-Brown G, Beilby JO, Tarbit MH. Venous changes in the endometrium of myomatous uteri. Obstet Gynecol 1971;38:743–51.
35. Wallach EE, Vlahos NF. Uterine myomas: an overview of development, clinical features, and management. Obstet Gynecol 2004;104:393–406.
36. Stewart EA, Nowak RA. Leiomyoma-related bleeding: a classic hypothesis updated for the molecular era. Hum Reprod Update 1996;2:295–306.
37. Lippman SA, Warner M, Samuels S, et al. Uterine fibroids and gynecologic pain symptoms in a population-based study. Fertil Steril 2003;80:1488–94.
38. Grover SR, Quinn MA. Is there any value in bimanual pelvic examination as a screening test. Med J Aust 1995;162:408–10.
39. Bansal T, Mehrotra P, Jayasena D, et al. Obstructive nephropathy and chronic kidney disease secondary to uterine leiomyomas. Arch Gynecol Obstet 2009;279:785–8.
40. Bukulmez O, Doody KJ. Clinical features of myomas. Obstet Gynecol Clin North Am 2006;33:69–84.

41. Practice Committee of American Society for Reproductive Medicine in collaboration with Society of Reproductive Surgeons. Myomas and reproductive function. Fertil Steril 2008;90:S125–30.
42. Pritts EA. Fibroids and infertility: a systematic review of the evidence. Obstet Gynecol Surv 2001;56:483–91.
43. Pritts EA, Parker WH, Olive DL. Fibroids and infertility: an updated systematic review of the evidence. Fertil Steril 2009;91:1215–23.
44. Levens ED, Wesley R, Premkumar A, et al. Magnetic resonance imaging and transvaginal ultrasound for determining fibroid burden: implications for research and clinical care. Am J Obstet Gynecol 2009;200:537.e1–7.
45. Cicinelli E, Romano F, Anastasio PS, et al. Transabdominal sonohysterography, transvaginal sonography, and hysteroscopy in the evaluation of submucous myomas. Obstet Gynecol 1995;85:42–7.
46. Griffin KW, Ellis MR, Wilder L, et al. Clinical inquiries. What is the appropriate diagnostic evaluation of fibroids? J Fam Pract 2005;54:458, 460, 462.
47. Dueholm M, Lundorf E, Hansen ES, et al. Accuracy of magnetic resonance imaging and transvaginal ultrasonography in the diagnosis, mapping, and measurement of uterine myomas. Am J Obstet Gynecol 2002;186:409–15.
48. Becker E Jr, Lev-Toaff AS, Kaufman EP, et al. The added value of transvaginal sonohysterography over transvaginal sonography alone in women with known or suspected leiomyoma. J Ultrasound Med 2002;21:237–47.
49. Volkers NA, Hehenkamp WJ, Spijkerboer AM, et al. MR reproducibility in the assessment of uterine fibroids for patients scheduled for uterine artery embolization. Cardiovasc Intervent Radiol 2008;31:260–8.
50. Dueholm M, Lundorf E, Hansen ES, et al. Evaluation of the uterine cavity with magnetic resonance imaging, transvaginal sonography, hysterosonographic examination, and diagnostic hysteroscopy. Fertil Steril 2001;76:350–7.
51. Dueholm M, Lundorf E, Sorensen JS, et al. Reproducibility of evaluation of the uterus by transvaginal sonography, hysterosonographic examination, hysteroscopy and magnetic resonance imaging. Hum Reprod 2002;17: 195–200.
52. Dudiak CM, Turner DA, Patel SK, et al. Uterine leiomyomas in the infertile patient: preoperative localization with MR imaging versus US and hysterosalpingography. Radiology 1988;167:627–30.
53. Vitiello D, McCarthy S. Diagnostic imaging of myomas. Obstet Gynecol Clin North Am 2006;33:85–95.
54. Mayer DP, Shipilov V. Ultrasonography and magnetic resonance imaging of uterine fibroids. Obstet Gynecol Clin North Am 1995;22:667–725.
55. Ascher SM, Arnold LL, Patt RH, et al. Adenomyosis: prospective comparison of MR imaging and transvaginal sonography. Radiology 1994;190:803–6.
56. Togashi K, Ozasa H, Konishi I, et al. Enlarged uterus: differentiation between adenomyosis and leiomyoma with MR imaging. Radiology 1989;171:531–4.
57. Schwartz LB, Zawin M, Carcangiu ML, et al. Does pelvic magnetic resonance imaging differentiate among the histologic subtypes of uterine leiomyomata? Fertil Steril 1998;70:580–7.
58. Deligdisch L, Hirschmann S, Altchek A. Pathologic changes in gonadotropin releasing hormone agonist analogue treated uterine leiomyomata. Fertil Steril 1997;67:837–41.
59. Lethaby A, Vollenhoven B, Sowter M. Pre-operative GnRH analogue therapy before hysterectomy or myomectomy for uterine fibroids. Cochrane Database Syst Rev 2000;(2):CD000547.

60. Tropeano G, Amoroso S, Scambia G. Non-surgical management of uterine fibroids. Hum Reprod Update 2008;14:259–74.
61. Spitz IM. Clinical utility of progesterone receptor modulators and their effect on the endometrium. Curr Opin Obstet Gynecol 2009;21:318–24.
62. Chwalisz K, Larsen L, Mattia-Goldberg C, et al. A randomized, controlled trial of asoprisnil, a novel selective progesterone receptor modulator, in women with uterine leiomyomata. Fertil Steril 2007;87:1399–412.
63. Levens ED, Potlog-Nahari C, Armstrong AY, et al. CDB-2914 for uterine leiomyomata treatment: a randomized controlled trial. Obstet Gynecol 2008;111: 1129–36.
64. Nieman LK, Blocker W, Nansel T, et al. Efficacy and tolerability of CDB-2914 treatment for symptomatic uterine fibroids: a randomized, double-blind, placebo-controlled, phase IIb study. Fertil Steril 2011;95:767–72.e1-2.
65. Donnez J, Tatarchuk TF, Bouchard P, et al. Ulipristal acetate versus placebo for fibroid treatment before surgery. N Engl J Med 2012;366:409–20.
66. Mutter GL, Bergeron C, Deligdisch L, et al. The spectrum of endometrial pathology induced by progesterone receptor modulators. Mod Pathol 2008;21: 591–8.
67. Howell A, Cuzick J, Baum M, et al. Results of the ATAC (Arimidex, Tamoxifen, Alone or in Combination) trial after completion of 5 years' adjuvant treatment for breast cancer. Lancet 2005;365:60–2.
68. Bulun SE, Simpson ER, Word RA. Expression of the CYP19 gene and its product aromatase cytochrome P450 in human uterine leiomyoma tissues and cells in culture. J Clin Endocrinol Metab 1994;78:736–43.
69. Ishikawa H, Reierstad S, Demura M, et al. High aromatase expression in uterine leiomyoma tissues of African-American women. J Clin Endocrinol Metab 2009;94: 1752–6.
70. Gurates B, Parmaksiz C, Kilic G, et al. Treatment of symptomatic uterine leiomyoma with letrozole. Reprod Biomed Online 2008;17:569–74.
71. Hilario SG, Bozzini N, Borsari R, et al. Action of aromatase inhibitor for treatment of uterine leiomyoma in perimenopausal patients. Fertil Steril 2009;91:240–3.
72. Kaunitz AM. Aromatase inhibitor therapy for uterine bleeding in a postmenopausal woman with leiomyomata. Menopause 2007;14:941–3.
73. Song H, Lu D, Navaratnam K, et al. Aromatase inhibitors for uterine fibroids. Cochrane Database Syst Rev 2013;(10):CD009505.
74. Zapata LB, Whiteman MK, Tepper NK, et al. Intrauterine device use among women with uterine fibroids: a systematic review. Contraception 2010;82:41–55.
75. Khan AT, Shehmar M, Gupta JK. Uterine fibroids: current perspectives. Int J Womens Health 2014;6:95–114.
76. American College of Obstetricians and Gynecologists. ACOG practice bulletin. Alternatives to hysterectomy in the management of leiomyomas. Obstet Gynecol 2008;112:387–400.
77. Hehenkamp WJ, Volkers NA, Birnie E, et al. Symptomatic uterine fibroids: treatment with uterine artery embolization or hysterectomy–results from the randomized clinical Embolisation versus Hysterectomy (EMMY) Trial. Radiology 2008; 246:823–32.
78. Moss JG, Cooper KG, Khaund A, et al. Randomised comparison of uterine artery embolisation (UAE) with surgical treatment in patients with symptomatic uterine fibroids (REST trial): 5-year results. BJOG 2011;118:936–44.
79. Gupta JK, Sinha AS, Lumsden MA, et al. Uterine artery embolization for symptomatic uterine fibroids. Cochrane Database Syst Rev 2006;(1):CD005073.

80. Walker WJ, Carpenter TT, Kent AS. Persistent vaginal discharge after uterine artery embolization for fibroid tumors: cause of the condition, magnetic resonance imaging appearance, and surgical treatment. Am J Obstet Gynecol 2004;190: 1230–3.

81. Pron G, Bennett J, Common A, et al. The Ontario Uterine Fibroid Embolization Trial. Part 2. Uterine fibroid reduction and symptom relief after uterine artery embolization for fibroids. Fertil Steril 2003;79:120–7.

82. Hehenkamp WJ, Volkers NA, Broekmans FJ, et al. Loss of ovarian reserve after uterine artery embolization: a randomized comparison with hysterectomy. Hum Reprod 2007;22:1996–2005.

83. Mara M, Maskova J, Fucikova Z, et al. Midterm clinical and first reproductive results of a randomized controlled trial comparing uterine fibroid embolization and myomectomy. Cardiovasc Intervent Radiol 2008;31:73–85.

84. Goldberg J, Pereira L, Berghella V, et al. Pregnancy outcomes after treatment for fibromyomata: uterine artery embolization versus laparoscopic myomectomy. Am J Obstet Gynecol 2004;191:18–21.

85. Pron G, Mocarski E, Bennett J, et al. Pregnancy after uterine artery embolization for leiomyomata: the Ontario multicenter trial. Obstet Gynecol 2005;105:67–76.

86. Clark NA, Mumford SL, Segars JH. Reproductive impact of MRI-guided focused ultrasound surgery for fibroids: a systematic review of the evidence. Curr Opin Obstet Gynecol 2014;26:151–61.

87. Behera MA, Leong M, Johnson L, et al. Eligibility and accessibility of magnetic resonance-guided focused ultrasound (MRgFUS) for the treatment of uterine leiomyomas. Fertil Steril 2010;94:1864–8.

88. Smart OC, Hindley JT, Regan L, et al. Gonadotrophin-releasing hormone and magnetic-resonance-guided ultrasound surgery for uterine leiomyomata. Obstet Gynecol 2006;108:49–54.

89. Gizzo S, Saccardi C, Patrelli TS, et al. Magnetic resonance-guided focused ultrasound myomectomy: safety, efficacy, subsequent fertility and quality-of-life improvements, a systematic review. Reprod Sci 2014;21:465–76.

90. Ringold S. FDA approves ultrasound fibroid therapy. JAMA 2004;292:2826.

91. Segars J. Fibroids. Chichester (West Sussex): John Wiley & Sons; 2013.

92. Camanni M, Bonino L, Delpiano EM, et al. Hysteroscopic management of large symptomatic submucous uterine myomas. J Minim Invasive Gynecol 2010;17: 59–65.

93. Griffin L, Feinglass J, Garrett A, et al. Postoperative outcomes after robotic versus abdominal myomectomy. JSLS 2013;17:407–13.

94. Sesti F, Cosi V, Calonzi F, et al. Randomized comparison of total laparoscopic, laparoscopically assisted vaginal and vaginal hysterectomies for myomatous uteri. Arch Gynecol Obstet 2014;290:485–91.

95. ACOG Releases Special Report on Power Morcellation and Occult Malignancy in Gynecologic Surgery. 2014. Available at: http://www.acog.org/About-ACOG/News-Room/News-Releases/2014/ACOG-Releases-Special-Report-on-Power-Morcellation-and-Occult-Malignancy-in-Gynecologic-Surgery. Accessed August 28, 2014.

96. Halder SK, Goodwin JS, Al-Hendy A. 1,25-Dihydroxyvitamin D3 reduces TGF-beta3-induced fibrosis-related gene expression in human uterine leiomyoma cells. J Clin Endocrinol Metab 2011;96:E754–62.

97. Zhang D, Al-Hendy M, Richard-Davis G, et al. Antiproliferative and proapoptotic effects of epigallocatechin gallate on human leiomyoma cells. Fertil Steril 2010; 94:1887–93.

98. Malik M, Mendoza M, Payson M, et al. Curcumin, a nutritional supplement with antineoplastic activity, enhances leiomyoma cell apoptosis and decreases fibronectin expression. Fertil Steril 2009;91:2177–84.
99. Catherino WH, Malik M. Uterine leiomyomas express a molecular pattern that lowers retinoic acid exposure. Fertil Steril 2007;87:1388–98.

Current Strategies for Endometriosis Management

Pinar H. Kodaman, MD, PhD

KEYWORDS

- Endometriosis • Laparoscopy • Endometrioma • Pelvic pain • Infertility

KEY POINTS

- There are several medical approaches to the management of endometriosis, all of which are fairly comparable in efficacy.
- Surgical evaluation is useful for the diagnosis of endometriosis, when medical treatments fail, and to enhance fertility.
- Endometriomas causing pain or those greater than 4 cm should be treated surgically, but damage to the ovary during cystectomy should be minimized.
- Fertility treatments in the setting of endometriosis should be based on stage of disease, age, and other factors that affect fecundity.

INTRODUCTION

Endometriosis, the presence of endometrial glands and stroma outside of the endometrial cavity, represents one of the most challenging gynecologic conditions to manage given its insidious onset, surgical diagnosis, association with pelvic pain and infertility, and often progressive nature. Endometriosis is a chronic disease affecting at least 10% of reproductive-aged women, but is found in approximately 40% of infertile women[1] and up to 90% of women with pelvic pain.[2] Risk factors include family history, low body mass index, alcohol use, smoking, particularly in the setting of infertility, Caucasian race, prolonged estrogen exposure as with early menarche or late menopause, and nutritional/environmental factors.[1,3,4]

The classic triad of endometriosis symptoms, dysmenorrhea, dyspareunia, and dyschezia, raises clinical suspicion for this disorder. However, the substantial overlap of endometriosis symptoms with other conditions causing pelvic pain, both

No conflicts of interest/nothing to disclose.
Department of Obstetrics, Gynecology, and Reproductive Sciences, Yale University School of Medicine, 333 Cedar Street, PO Box 208063, New Haven, CT 06520-8063, USA
E-mail address: pinar.kodaman@yale.edu

Obstet Gynecol Clin N Am 42 (2015) 87–101
http://dx.doi.org/10.1016/j.ogc.2014.10.005
0889-8545/15/$ – see front matter © 2015 Elsevier Inc. All rights reserved.

gynecologic and nongynecologic, combined with the limitation of pelvic examination in detecting endometriosis, makes clinical diagnosis challenging. Furthermore, the amount of endometriosis present does not necessarily correlate with symptoms,[5] and therefore, the usefulness of available staging systems is limited.[6] Ultimately, surgical intervention is required for confirmation of endometriosis, and this, in part, contributes to the delayed diagnosis of this disorder, sometimes over a decade, particularly in the younger population,[7,8] wherein conservative, nonsurgical interventions tend to be prolonged. Whether such delayed diagnosis affects the progression of the disease and its long-term sequelae, such as infertility, remains unclear.

The challenging nature of endometriosis, in part, stems from a still limited understanding of its pathophysiology. Various theories have been proposed for its development, including retrograde menstruation, coelomic metaplasia, and lymphatic or hematologic spread.[9] More recently, stem cells have been implicated in the pathogenesis of endometriosis[10]; however, no one theory to date is sufficient to explain all of the clinical findings and features of the disorder. For example, although 90% of women have retrograde menstruation, only a small fraction of these women develop endometriosis.[11] There appears to be a peritoneal predisposition to the attachment and survival of endometriosis implants in some women and not in others.[12]

The different proposed pathophysiologic mechanisms may help explain the varied endometriosis phenotypes, including superficial peritoneal endometriosis implants, deep infiltrating endometriosis (DIE), endometriomas, and adenomyosis. Although much less common, endometriosis can also present outside of the pelvis, as seen with pleural, nasal, intrahepatic, diaphragmatic, and abdominal wall endometriosis.[13–15] With respect to abdominal wall endometriosis, which is the most common form of extrapelvic endometriosis, the pain is not necessarily cyclic and is associated with a mass in the abdominal wall, most frequently at the site of a previous incision. In general, catamenial symptoms, regardless of location, should raise suspicion for the presence of endometriosis.

Medical and surgical treatments are mainstays in the management of endometriosis, and different approaches are dictated by the pleiotropic manifestations of the disease as well as underlying patient characteristics. In general, medical treatment options are limited when fertility is desired because of the ovarian suppression inherent in their mechanisms of action. Assisted reproductive technologies can often overcome the detrimental effects of endometriosis without prerequisite surgical intervention. This review focuses on current strategies for the management of endometriosis in the setting of pain and infertility.

ENDOMETRIOSIS AND PAIN

As mentioned above, endometriosis is found in most women with pelvic pain,[2] both chronic and cyclic, and thus should be strongly considered in the differential diagnosis of pelvic pain, while keeping in mind other nongynecologic causes, which may coexist or represent sole causes for such symptoms. There are various manifestations of endometriosis, including endometriomas, adenomyosis, dark or red lesions, clear vesicles, peritoneal windows, and powder burns, each of which may cause pain by different mechanisms.[16] Pain can arise from cyclic bleeding from ectopic endometrial tissue, production of inflammatory mediators, such as cytokines, and nerve irritation.[16] The most severe pain is associated with deep (>6 mm) invasion of the peritoneum[17] as seen with DIE, which is frequently found in the obliterated cul-de-sac.[18] In addition, pelvic adhesions from the inflammation that occurs with endometriosis can also contribute to pelvic pain.

MEDICAL TREATMENT OF ENDOMETRIOSIS

The medical treatment options for endometriosis rely on the suppression of endometriosis by manipulating the hormonal milieu because endometriosis growth and activation are stimulated by estrogen, and both estrogen and progesterone receptors are present in ectopic endometrial tissue.[17] Although controlling the pain and potentially the progression of endometriosis, such hormonal manipulation also contributes to the side effects of these medical treatments.

Nonhormonal-based treatments, such as nonsteroidal anti-inflammatory drugs, are helpful in the management of primary dysmenorrhea; however, they do not significantly improve endometriosis pain.[19] The use of narcotics for the treatment of endometriosis pain will not be addressed in depth, although it is important to note that treatment of chronic pelvic pain due to endometriosis requires a multidisciplinary approach, and narcotics may sometimes be indicated for long-term control of symptoms or transiently during the perioperative period.

The available hormonal options, which are discussed later, have similar efficacies, and therefore, can be interchanged should bothersome side effects ensue. It should be noted, however, that there is an approximately 40% placebo effect in the treatment of pelvic pain[20] that should be factored into the evaluation of treatment success. **Box 1** lists the available medical treatment options for endometriosis-related pelvic pain.

Combined Hormonal Contraceptives

Hormonal contraceptives containing both ethinyl estradiol (EE) and progestin can be used in a cyclic or continuous fashion for the treatment of endometriosis. Continuous use appears to result in better pain control,[21] and such a regimen may make combined hormonal contraceptives (CHCs) more comparable to GnRH analogues, which also result in amenorrhea. Although direct comparative studies of extended use CHC and GnRH analogues are lacking, cyclic CHC use compares favorably with GnRH analogues in treating dyspareunia and noncyclic pelvic pain.[22]

Although CHCs containing older, androgenic progestins have been preferred in the treatment of endometriosis, the newer generation progestins also appear to have good efficacy.[23] Although low-dose EE containing pills have been advocated because of the known proliferative actions of estrogen on endometriosis, EE appears to potentiate the antiproliferative effects of progestin by inducing progesterone receptors expression in vitro.[24] The optimal EE dose in CHC for endometriosis has not been defined, and therefore, selection of CHC should be based on side-effect profile and underlying patient characteristics, such as age, medical conditions, smoking status, and family history. The progestin component of CHC results in decidualization with subsequent atrophy of the eutopic endometrium and also appears to have several other mechanisms of action, including inhibition of matrix metalloproteases,[25] which promote invasion of ectopic endometrial tissue, and antiangiogenic effects.[26]

Box 1
Available medical treatments for endometriosis

Combined hormonal contraceptives (cyclic or continuous)

Progestin-only contraceptives (oral, injectable, implantable, intrauterine)

GnRH agonists

Aromatase inhibitors (in conjunction with ovarian suppression in premenopausal woman)

Danazol

Progestin-only Contraceptives

Both long-acting and short-acting progestins are effective in the treatment of endometriosis. These long-acting and short-acting progestins include medroxyprogesterone acetate (MPA) in daily or depot form, the implantable etonogestrel-containing rod, and other 19-nortestosterone derivatives, such as norethindrone and levonorgestrel. With respect to the latter, the levonorgestrel-releasing intrauterine system (LNG-IUS) represents a newer treatment option for endometriosis, which minimizes systemic side effects due to its mostly localized actions. Typical side effects of progestin-only contraceptives include erratic bleeding, weight gain, and mood symptoms. However, pain reduction is in the range of 70% to 100%, and therefore, patient satisfaction and compliance in the setting of endometriosis are good.[27] With progestin-only contraceptives, the typical continuous administration results in high rates of amenorrhea, and this likely contributes to pain control.

Levonorgestrel-releasing Intrauterine System

Recent data from several studies support the use of the LNG-IUS as a first-line treatment option for the medical management of endometriosis as well as for postsurgical control of recurrence.[28–30] In particular, a randomized controlled trial (RCT) comparing LNG-IUS to GnRH analogue found similar efficacy in the control of endometriosis-related pain.[31] A recent meta-analysis concurred with this finding and, in addition, emphasized the favorable side-effect profile of LNG-IUS compared with GnRH analogues, which cause bone loss and other hypoestrogenic effects.[32] LNG-IUS also has a beneficial effect on lipid profile, such that total and low-density lipoprotein cholesterol levels are decreased with no change in high-density lipoprotein cholesterol levels.[32]

There are also data to support the use of LNG-IUS for rectovaginal endometriosis[33] and adenomyosis,[34] with significant improvement in dyspareunia, bleeding, and pain. Although LNG-IUS only suppresses 25% to 50% of ovulations after the first 3 months of use,[35] it nevertheless appears to prevent recurrence of endometriomas following surgical resection comparable to CHCs (4.8% vs 10.5%, respectively).[36] Potential mechanisms for this include the atrophy of eutopic endometrium and subsequent reduction of retrograde menstruation as well as the high local concentrations of levonorgestrel in the peritoneal cavity, which may have direct inhibitory effects on ovarian endometrioma formation.[35]

Etonogestrel

There are limited, but promising data for the use of the implantable etonogestrel rod in the treatment of endometriosis-related pain as it has a known beneficial effect on dysmenorrhea.[37] A recent RCT demonstrated a significant decrease in pain by 68% after 6 months of use compared with 54% in the MPA group, and patient satisfaction in both groups was about 60%.[38] Although like MPA, etonogestrel has the frequent side effect of breakthrough bleeding, it may be preferable to MPA in the setting of elevated body mass index[39] and has the additional advantage of 3 years of ovarian suppression after subdermal implantation.

Other Progestins and Antiprogestins

Several studies now demonstrate that the progestin dienogest improves pelvic pain in the setting of endometriosis[40–42] with persistent beneficial effects for 6 months after discontinuation.[42] In addition, although dienogest is a 19-nortestosterone derivative, it lacks the androgenic side effects common to others in this group.[43] Unfortunately, although dienogest is widely used in Europe, Australia, and Japan, it is not available in the United States.[39] Similarly, the antiprogestins gestrinone and mifepristone are also not approved for use, but represent potential alternative medical treatments for endometriosis via a progestational withdrawal effect.[25,44]

Gonadotropin-releasing Agonists

Despite significant hypoestrogenic side effects, gonadotropin-releasing agonists (GnRHa) therapy, in injectable or nasal spray form, remains a mainstay in the treatment of endometriosis due to reliable ovarian suppression. A large meta-analysis demonstrated that GnRHa improves endometriosis-related pain by 60% to 100%.[45] This favorable response to GnRHa does not efficiently diagnose endometriosis because a similar effect on pelvic pain, dysmenorrhea, and dyspareunia is observed even among women who do not have endometriosis.[46] Nevertheless, GnRHa can be used empirically to treat presumed endometriosis or postoperatively to delay recurrence of disease.[47]

Add-back therapy to minimize bone loss and to help control other hypoestrogenic side effects, such as hot flashes and vaginal dryness, should be started at the initiation of GnRHa therapy. Without such add-back, bone loss with GnRHa is 13% after 6 months.[48] Although norethindrone acetate is the only US Food and Drug Administration–approved add-back therapy, low-dose estrogen or a combination of low-dose estrogen and progestin can be used based on the hypothesis that there is a threshold for estrogen below which endometriosis is not stimulated.[49]

Injectable GnRH antagonists have a quicker onset of action in the suppression of the hypothalamic pituitary ovarian axis compared with GnRHa and can be used in the treatment of endometriosis[50]; however, data are limited, and the current cost of these medications is prohibitive for long-term ovarian suppression. They can be used transiently during the initiation of GnRHa to bypass the flare effect of the latter. A few days of overlap is sufficient and can be particularly useful when GnRHa needs to be initiated in the follicular phase of the menstrual cycle. Although not yet available for clinical use, the oral GnRH antagonist elagolix appears to have promise in the treatment of endometriosis-associated pain with minimal effect on bone loss.[51,52]

Aromatase Inhibitors

The synthesis of estrogen is blocked by aromatase inhibitors, which are, as a result, effective at decreasing pelvic pain due to endometriosis.[53,54] Aromatase inhibitors are as effective as GnRH in treating adenomyosis as well.[55] In premenopausal women, aromatase inhibitors must be used in conjunction with ovarian suppression because ovulation induction (OI) is otherwise a problematic side effect. In postmenopausal women, aromatase inhibitors can treat the gonadotropin-independent local estrogen production by ectopic endometriosis implants, which can persist after both natural and surgical menopause.[56,57] Limitations of aromatase inhibitors include negative effects on bone, off-label use, and unknown long-term effects. The combination of CHCs and aromatase inhibitors may abrogate bone loss in premenopausal women with endometriosis.[54]

Danazol

The 17α-ethinyl testosterone derivative danazol blocks ovarian steroidogenesis, but its use is limited by its androgenic side effects, such as acne, hirsutism, and voice deepening.[56,58] Although less well-tolerated than GnRHa, danazol provides similar pain relief[59] and therefore can be considered when other options are not viable.

SURGICAL TREATMENT OF ENDOMETRIOSIS

Although surgical evaluation is required for the definitive diagnosis of endometriosis, it can also be used to manage pelvic pain refractory to medical therapies and has a role in the treatment of infertility, which is discussed in the next section. Laparoscopy is the standard of care for the surgical management of endometriosis, and the objectives of such surgery include optimal treatment of all visible and deep disease, restoration of normal anatomy, and adhesion prevention.[60,61] A large meta-analysis shows that operative laparoscopy improves pain in 100%, 70%, and 40% of women with moderate, mild, and minimal endometriosis, respectively,[62] and pain recurrence ranges from 20% to 40% after both initial and subsequent surgeries.[63] Repeated surgeries should be avoided when possible because of risks of surgery, including postoperative adhesions, and a decrease in ovarian reserve with iatrogenic ovarian damage.[56]

Based on a recent meta-analysis, there is no clear superiority of excision versus ablation for the surgical management of endometriosis[64]; however, excision allows for histologic diagnosis and removal of deeper lesions that may have a superficial appearance. It is for these reasons that many advocate excision of endometriosis lesions whenever possible.[60,65]

Preoperative Imaging

Given the limitations of physical examination findings in the detection of endometriosis, imaging is often indicated, particularly preoperatively for surgical planning. Transvaginal ultrasound (TVUS) is the first-line imaging modality for endometriosis because it is excellent at visualizing the female reproductive tract, cheaper than MRI, and widely available, including in the office setting.[60,66] Although basic TVUS is good for evaluating endometriomas and adenomyosis, it has limitations in the detection of bowel endometriosis and obliteration of the cul-de-sac.[67] These limitations can be overcome through the addition of adjuvant measures, including bowel preparation with enema before TVUS[68,69] or use of the visceral sliding sign, which looks for free movement of the anterior rectosigmoid relative to the posterior uterus in real-time.[70] Such modified TVUS techniques increase the diagnostic sensitivity and specificity to a level comparable to that of MRI.[71] More recently, transrectal ultrasonography has been evaluated for the diagnosis of bowel involvement by DIE; however, while muscularis infiltration can be detected, visualization of lesions involving the mucosal layer remains limited as with other diagnostic imaging modalities.[72,73] Nevertheless, because the need for bowel surgery is 3-fold greater in women with an obliterated cul-de-sac, preoperative evaluation of this area is essential.[74]

Surgical Management of Deep Infiltrating Endometriosis

Optimal surgical debulking of DIE requires careful surgical planning, including preoperative bowel preparation. If DIE involves bowel, which affects 3.8% to 37% of women with endometriosis,[75] bowel resection may be required, including superficial discoid resection or segmental bowel resection with anastomosis. Although incompletely resected DIE can be managed with postoperative GnRHa treatment,[76] preoperative diagnosis of DIE should prompt referral of the patient to a center capable of managing such advanced disease to avoid incomplete treatment, which will result in earlier recurrence[60] and need for repeat surgeries.

Surgical Management of Endometrioma

Medical management of endometriomas can result in the stabilization of cyst size and/or temporary shrinkage, but definitive surgical therapy is required when endometriomas remain symptomatic or large.[56,77] Even when asymptomatic, endometriomas greater than 4 cm may necessitate surgical intervention for histopathologic diagnosis given the association of endometriomas with endometrioid and clear cell ovarian cancers.[78] Although cystectomy for endometriomas can diminish ovarian reserve as measured by postoperative anti-Müllerian hormone (AMH) levels,[79] it does not appear to impair response to OI,[80] and for endometriomas greater than 4 cm, cystectomy improves fertility outcomes compared with coagulation or drainage.[77,81] In addition, excisional surgery for endometriomas is superior to ablation or drainage because of a high risk of recurrence with the latter procedures.[77] The use of a hybrid surgical procedure involving excision of most of the endometrioma and coagulation of the portion at the hilus may minimize ovarian tissue damage and preserve vascularization to the ovary.[82] However, a recent study shows that AMH decreases significantly regardless of the surgical approach for endometrioma.[83]

Presacral Neurectomy

Presacral neurectomy (PSN) is a technically difficult procedure involving excision of a portion of the superior hypogastric plexus that provides sympathetic innervation to the uterus. It can be considered for women with central pelvic pain and endometriosis/adenomyosis, particularly if they desire uterine preservation.[56] Although laparoscopic uterosacral nerve ablation appears to have no benefit based on large RCT,[84] PSN has a beneficial effect on long-term pain control compared with conservative laparoscopic surgery alone.[85]

Hysterectomy

Hysterectomy with bilateral salpingo-oophorectomy (BSO) represents definitive surgical management for endometriosis and has the lowest risk of disease recurrence as long as optimal debulking is achieved.[60] There is, however, a 10% to 15% risk of pain persistence and 3% to 5% risk of worsening pain with time.[63] Unilateral or bilateral ovarian preservation at the time of hysterectomy can be considered for younger women,[60] but carries a 6-fold higher risk of reoperation compared with women who have undergone BSO.[63] When performing a hysterectomy/BSO after completion of child-bearing, one should take into consideration the risks of surgical menopause, including detrimental effects on cardiovascular and bone health.[56] Hormone therapy (HT) will be required in the younger woman and should include progestin-only or combined HT to prevent the proliferative effects of unopposed estrogen on microscopic or residual disease.[56] Based on one RCT, the risk of recurrent endometriosis with combined HT use is only 3.5%.[86]

ENDOMETRIOSIS AND INFERTILITY

Although 30% to 50% of infertile women have endometriosis, the reverse is also true, such that 30% to 50% of women with endometriosis have infertility.[1] Endometriosis may affect fertility by various mechanisms, including distortion of pelvic anatomy from adhesions, intraperitoneal inflammation, which can decrease oocyte quality and/or oocyte-sperm interactions, abnormal tubal transport, and implantation defects.[87]

   Laparoscopic excision of endometriosis may have a beneficial effect on subsequent fertility[88]; however, there is no role for the medical management of endometriosis in the setting of infertility with the exception of 3 to 6 months of pretreatment with GnRH analogue before IVF, which appears to increase live birth rates.[89] Other forms of ovarian suppression before fertility treatments, such as CHC and danazol, do not improve pregnancy or live birth outcomes.[90]

OI/intrauterine insemination (IUI) using clomiphene citrate (CC) for endometriosis is more likely to result in pregnancy than timed intercourse alone (9.5% vs 3.3%)[91]; however, CC is not as effective as gonadotropins.[92] A large meta-analysis demonstrated that women with endometriosis have significantly decreased pregnancy rates following in vitro fertilization (IVF) compared with women with tubal factor infertility[93]; nevertheless, IVF remains the most effective fertility treatment for endometriosis,[87] with a cumulative live birth rate greater than 60% after 4 cycles.[94]

Because of age-related decreases in ovarian reserve and oocyte quality, the approach to the treatment of infertility in the setting of endometriosis should be based on age of the woman in addition to other coexisting infertility factors, if present. For example, if there is a surgically modifiable tubal factor, surgical intervention may be a good option, whereas with significant male factor, directly proceeding to IVF with intracytoplasmic sperm injection is the more reasonable approach. The stage of endometriosis also influences the choice of treatment for infertility (**Figs. 1** and **2**).

Stage I/II Endometriosis and Infertility

For early-stage endometriosis, laparoscopic excision or ablation has a small, but significant positive effect on subsequent spontaneous fertility; however, the number needed to treat is 12, and if endometriosis is not found at every diagnostic laparoscopy for suspected early-stage disease, the number needed to treat may be as high as 40, that is, 40 laparoscopies to achieve one additional pregnancy.[87,88] As a result, in asymptomatic women with possible early-stage endometriosis and normal ultrasound, laparoscopy is a low-yield intervention.[87]

On the other hand, OI/IUI with gonadotropins has been shown to increase the pregnancy rate among women with known stage I/II endometriosis (15% vs 4.5%

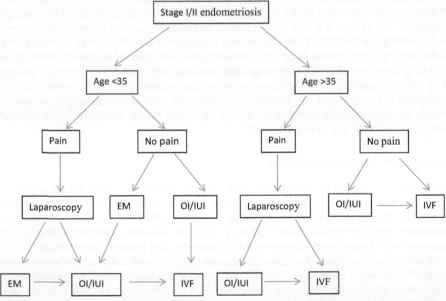

Fig. 1. Algorithm for treatment of infertility for presumed or known early-stage endometriosis. (*Data from* Revised American Society for Reproductive Medicine classification of endometriosis: 1996. Fertil Steril 1997;67(5):817–21.)

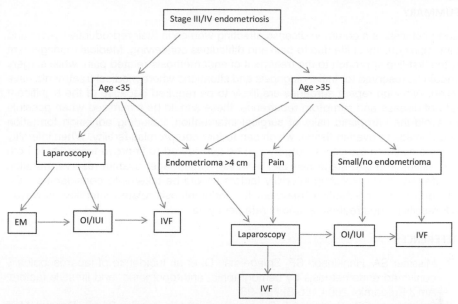

Fig. 2. Algorithm for treatment of infertility for presumed or known late-stage endometriosis. (*Data from* Revised American Society for Reproductive Medicine classification of endometriosis: 1996. Fertil Steril 1997;67(5):817–21.)

untreated),[92] and although the success rate of OI/IUI among women with undiagnosed, early endometriosis is unknown, similar per-cycle pregnancy and cumulative live birth rates (about 20% and 65%, respectively) are seen following 4 cycles of OI/IUI among women with unexplained infertility and that due to minimal or mild endometriosis.[95]

As **Fig. 1** shows, in asymptomatic women less than 35 years old, expectant management (EM) versus OI/IUI are reasonable initial treatment options. However, in symptomatic young women, laparoscopy for endometriosis will help with pain and increase fecundity; thus, surgery may be followed by EM or OI/IUI.[87] If OI/IUI is not successful, IVF is the next step (see **Fig. 1**). In the older (>35 years old) woman with stage I/II endometriosis, pain should prompt laparoscopic intervention followed by OI/IUI or IVF; however, one of the latter 2 treatments can be pursued directly if pain is not present (see **Fig. 1**).

Stage III/IV Endometriosis

As shown in **Fig. 2**, in advanced disease, pain regardless of age will also lead to surgical intervention as should large endometriomas (>4 cm), even if asymptomatic, for histopathologic confirmation, for easier access to ovaries for oocyte retrieval, and to prevent endometrioma rupture/leakage.[87] Endometrioma resection also appears to have a beneficial effect on IVF success rates.[81]

If pain or large endometriomas are not an issue in the older woman, a more aggressive approach with OI/IUI versus IVF without initial surgical intervention is recommended; however, in the younger woman with no other infertility factors, initial surgery can be considered an alternative to IVF.[87] Repeated surgeries are not helpful for infertility, and therefore, if initial surgical intervention fails to result in pregnancy, IVF should be pursued.[63,87]

SUMMARY

Endometriosis is a common disease affecting women in their reproductive years and can impair quality of life due to pain and difficulties conceiving. Medical management is the first-line approach to the treatment of endometriosis-related pain, while surgery should be reserved for initial diagnosis and situations where medical treatments have failed. Although repeat surgeries are likely to be required because of the significant rate of disease and symptom recurrence, these should be minimized when possible to avoid the iatrogenic risks of surgical intervention, including adhesion formation and damage to ovarian tissue, which can further compromise fertility. When infertility is the presenting symptom, surgery can be considered to improve fecundity in both early-stage and late-stage disease; however, patient age, ovarian reserve, duration of infertility, and coexisting infertility factors should be taken into consideration. OI/IUI represents an effective treatment for endometriosis-related infertility; however, IVF results in the greatest fecundity rate per cycle.

REFERENCES

1. Missmer SA, Hankinson SE, Spiegelman D, et al. Incidence of laparoscopically confirmed endometriosis by demographic, anthropometric, and lifestyle factors. Am J Epidemiol 2004;160(8):784–96.
2. Spaczynski RZ, Duleba AJ. Diagnosis of endometriosis. Semin Reprod Med 2003;21(2):193–208.
3. Hadfield RM, Mardon HJ, Barlow DH, et al. Endometriosis in monozygotic twins. Fertil Steril 1997;68(5):941–2.
4. Harris HR, Chavarro JE, Malspeis S, et al. Dairy-food, calcium, magnesium, and vitamin D intake and endometriosis: a prospective cohort study. Am J Epidemiol 2013;177(5):420–30.
5. Vercellini P, Trespidi L, De Giorgi O, et al. Endometriosis and pelvic pain: relation to disease stage and localization. Fertil Steril 1996;65(2):299–304.
6. Revised American Society for reproductive medicine classification of endometriosis: 1996. Fertil Steril 1997;67(5):817–21.
7. Hadfield R, Mardon H, Barlow D, et al. Delay in the diagnosis of endometriosis: a survey of women from the USA and the UK. Hum Reprod 1996;11(4):878–80.
8. Ballard K, Lowton K, Wright J. What's the delay? A qualitative study of women's experiences of reaching a diagnosis of endometriosis. Fertil Steril 2006;86(5):1296–301.
9. Sampson JA. Metastatic or embolic endometriosis, due to the menstrual dissemination of endometrial tissue into the venous circulation. Am J Pathol 1927;3(2):93–110.43.
10. Gargett CE, Schwab KE, Brosens JJ, et al. Potential role of endometrial stem/progenitor cells in the pathogenesis of early-onset endometriosis. Mol Hum Reprod 2014;20(7):591–8.
11. Halme J, Hammond MG, Hulka JF, et al. Retrograde menstruation in healthy women and in patients with endometriosis. Obstet Gynecol 1984;64(2):151–4.
12. Young VJ, Brown JK, Saunders PT, et al. The role of the peritoneum in the pathogenesis of endometriosis. Hum Reprod Update 2013;19(5):558–69.
13. Mignemi G, Facchini C, Raimondo D, et al. A case report of nasal endometriosis in a patient affected by Behcet's disease. J Minim Invasive Gynecol 2012;19(4):514–6.
14. Ecker AM, Donnellan NM, Shepherd JP, et al. Abdominal wall endometriosis: 12 years of experience at a large academic institution. Am J Obstet Gynecol 2014;211(4):363.e1–5.

15. Fluegen G, Jankowiak F, Zacarias Foehrding L, et al. Intrahepatic endometriosis as differential diagnosis: case report and literature review. World J Gastroenterol 2013;19(29):4818–22.
16. Howard FM. Endometriosis and mechanisms of pelvic pain. J Minim Invasive Gynecol 2009;16(5):540–50.
17. Donnez J, Nisolle M, Smoes P, et al. Peritoneal endometriosis and "endometriotic" nodules of the rectovaginal septum are two different entities. Fertil Steril 1996; 66(3):362–8.
18. Porpora MG, Koninckx PR, Piazze J, et al. Correlation between endometriosis and pelvic pain. J Am Assoc Gynecol Laparosc 1999;6(4):429–34.
19. Allen C, Hopewell S, Prentice A, et al. Nonsteroidal anti-inflammatory drugs for pain in women with endometriosis. Cochrane Database Syst Rev 2009;(2):CD004753.
20. Turner JA, Deyo RA, Loeser JD, et al. The importance of placebo effects in pain treatment and research. JAMA 1994;271(20):1609–14.
21. Vercellini P, Frontino G, De Giorgi O, et al. Continuous use of an oral contraceptive for endometriosis-associated recurrent dysmenorrhea that does not respond to a cyclic pill regimen. Fertil Steril 2003;80(3):560–3.
22. Vercellini P, Trespidi L, Colombo A, et al. A gonadotropin-releasing hormone agonist versus a low-dose oral contraceptive for pelvic pain associated with endometriosis. Fertil Steril 1993;60(1):75–9.
23. Razzi S, Luisi S, Ferretti C, et al. Use of a progestogen only preparation containing desogestrel in the treatment of recurrent pelvic pain after conservative surgery for endometriosis. Eur J Obstet Gynecol Reprod Biol 2007;135(2):188–90.
24. Bono Y, Kyo S, Kiyono T, et al. Concurrent estrogen action was essential for maximal progestin effect in oral contraceptives. Fertil Steril 2014;101(5):1337–43.
25. Olive DL. Medical therapy of endometriosis. Semin Reprod Med 2003;21(2): 209–22.
26. Laschke MW, Menger MD. Anti-angiogenic treatment strategies for the therapy of endometriosis. Hum Reprod Update 2012;18(6):682–702.
27. Vercellini P, Cortesi I, Crosignani PG. Progestins for symptomatic endometriosis: a critical analysis of the evidence. Fertil Steril 1997;68(3):393–401.
28. Abou-Setta AM, Houston B, Al-Inany HG, et al. Levonorgestrel-releasing intrauterine device (LNG-IUD) for symptomatic endometriosis following surgery. Cochrane Database Syst Rev 2013;(1):CD005072.
29. Lockhat FB, Emembolu JO, Konje JC. The efficacy, side-effects and continuation rates in women with symptomatic endometriosis undergoing treatment with an intra-uterine administered progestogen (levonorgestrel): a 3 year follow-up. Hum Reprod 2005;20(3):789–93.
30. Lockhat FB, Emembolu JO, Konje JC. The evaluation of the effectiveness of an intrauterine-administered progestogen (levonorgestrel) in the symptomatic treatment of endometriosis and in the staging of the disease. Hum Reprod 2004;19(1):179–84.
31. Petta CA, Ferriani RA, Abrao MS, et al. Randomized clinical trial of a levonorgestrel-releasing intrauterine system and a depot GnRH analogue for the treatment of chronic pelvic pain in women with endometriosis. Hum Reprod 2005;20(7):1993–8.
32. Lan S, Ling L, Jianhong Z, et al. Analysis of the levonorgestrel-releasing intrauterine system in women with endometriosis. J Int Med Res 2013;41(3):548–58.
33. Fedele L, Bianchi S, Zanconato G, et al. Use of a levonorgestrel-releasing intrauterine device in the treatment of rectovaginal endometriosis. Fertil Steril 2001; 75(3):485–8.

34. Kelekci S, Kelekci KH, Yilmaz B. Effects of levonorgestrel-releasing intrauterine system and T380A intrauterine copper device on dysmenorrhea and days of bleeding in women with and without adenomyosis. Contraception 2012;86(5):458–63.
35. Lockhat FB, Emembolu JE, Konje JC. Serum and peritoneal fluid levels of levonorgestrel in women with endometriosis who were treated with an intrauterine contraceptive device containing levonorgestrel. Fertil Steril 2005;83(2):398–404.
36. Cho S, Jung JA, Lee Y, et al. Postoperative levonorgestrel-releasing intrauterine system versus oral contraceptives after gonadotropin-releasing hormone agonist treatment for preventing endometrioma recurrence. Acta Obstet Gynecol Scand 2014;93(1):38–44.
37. Wenzl R, van Beek A, Schnabel P, et al. Pharmacokinetics of etonogestrel released from the contraceptive implant Implanon. Contraception 1998;58(5): 283–8.
38. Walch K, Unfried G, Huber J, et al. Implanon versus medroxyprogesterone acetate: effects on pain scores in patients with symptomatic endometriosis–a pilot study. Contraception 2009;79(1):29–34.
39. Angioni S, Cofelice V, Pontis A, et al. New trends of progestins treatment of endometriosis. Gynecol Endocrinol 2014;30(11):769–73.
40. Harada T, Momoeda M, Taketani Y, et al. Dienogest is as effective as intranasal buserelin acetate for the relief of pain symptoms associated with endometriosis–a randomized, double-blind, multicenter, controlled trial. Fertil Steril 2009; 91(3):675–81.
41. Strowitzki T, Faustmann T, Gerlinger C, et al. Dienogest in the treatment of endometriosis-associated pelvic pain: a 12-week, randomized, double-blind, placebo-controlled study. Eur J Obstet Gynecol Reprod Biol 2010;151(2):193–8.
42. Petraglia F, Hornung D, Seitz C, et al. Reduced pelvic pain in women with endometriosis: efficacy of long-term dienogest treatment. Arch Gynecol Obstet 2012; 285(1):167–73.
43. Ruan X, Seeger H, Mueck AO. The pharmacology of dienogest. Maturitas 2012; 71(4):337–44.
44. Brown J, Kives S, Akhtar M. Progestagens and anti-progestagens for pain associated with endometriosis. Cochrane Database Syst Rev 2012;(3): CD002122.
45. Prentice A, Deary AJ, Goldbeck-Wood S, et al. Gonadotrophin-releasing hormone analogues for pain associated with endometriosis. Cochrane Database Syst Rev 2000;(2):CD000346.
46. Ling FW. Randomized controlled trial of depot leuprolide in patients with chronic pelvic pain and clinically suspected endometriosis. Pelvic Pain Study Group. Obstet Gynecol 1999;93(1):51–8.
47. Vercellini P, Crosignani PG, Fadini R, et al. A gonadotrophin-releasing hormone agonist compared with expectant management after conservative surgery for symptomatic endometriosis. Br J Obstet Gynaecol 1999;106(7):672–7.
48. Al Kadri H, Hassan S, Al-Fozan HM, et al. Hormone therapy for endometriosis and surgical menopause. Cochrane Database Syst Rev 2009;(1):CD005997.
49. Barbieri RL. Endometriosis and the estrogen threshold theory. Relation to surgical and medical treatment. J Reprod Med 1998;43(3 Suppl):287–92.
50. Kupker W, Felberbaum RE, Krapp M, et al. Use of GnRH antagonists in the treatment of endometriosis. Reprod Biomed Online 2002;5(1):12–6.
51. Carr B, Dmowski WP, O'Brien C, et al. Elagolix, an oral GnRH antagonist, versus subcutaneous depot medroxyprogesterone acetate for the treatment of endometriosis: effects on bone mineral density. Reprod Sci 2014;21(11):1341–51.

52. Diamond MP, Carr B, Dmowski WP, et al. Elagolix treatment for endometriosis-associated pain: results from a phase 2, randomized, double-blind, placebo-controlled study. Reprod Sci 2014;21(3):363–71.
53. Nawathe A, Patwardhan S, Yates D, et al. Systematic review of the effects of aromatase inhibitors on pain associated with endometriosis. BJOG 2008;115(7): 818–22.
54. Pavone ME, Bulun SE. Aromatase inhibitors for the treatment of endometriosis. Fertil Steril 2012;98(6):1370–9.
55. Badawy AM, Elnashar AM, Mosbah AA. Aromatase inhibitors or gonadotropin-releasing hormone agonists for the management of uterine adenomyosis: a randomized controlled trial. Acta Obstet Gynecol Scand 2012;91(4):489–95.
56. Treatment of pelvic pain associated with endometriosis: a committee opinion. Fertil Steril 2014;101(4):927–35.
57. Polyzos NP, Fatemi HM, Zavos A, et al. Aromatase inhibitors in post-menopausal endometriosis. Reprod Biol Endocrinol 2011;9:90.
58. Selak V, Farquhar C, Prentice A, et al. Danazol for pelvic pain associated with endometriosis. Cochrane Database Syst Rev 2007;(4):CD000068.
59. Brown J, Pan A, Hart RJ. Gonadotrophin-releasing hormone analogues for pain associated with endometriosis. Cochrane Database Syst Rev 2010;(12): CD008475.
60. Yeung P Jr. The laparoscopic management of endometriosis in patients with pelvic pain. Obstet Gynecol Clin North Am 2014;41(3):371–83.
61. Johnson NP, Hummelshoj L. Consensus on current management of endometriosis. Hum Reprod 2013;28(6):1552–68.
62. Jacobson TZ, Duffy JM, Barlow D, et al. Laparoscopic surgery for pelvic pain associated with endometriosis. Cochrane Database Syst Rev 2009;(4):CD001300.
63. Berlanda N, Vercellini P, Fedele L. The outcomes of repeat surgery for recurrent symptomatic endometriosis. Curr Opin Obstet Gynecol 2010;22(4):320–5.
64. Duffy JM, Arambage K, Correa FJ, et al. Laparoscopic surgery for endometriosis. Cochrane Database Syst Rev 2014;(4):CD011031.
65. Garry R. The effectiveness of laparoscopic excision of endometriosis. Curr Opin Obstet Gynecol 2004;16(4):299–303.
66. Exacoustos C, Manganaro L, Zupi E. Imaging for the evaluation of endometriosis and adenomyosis. Best Pract Res Clin Obstet Gynaecol 2014;28(5):655–81.
67. Brosens I, Puttemans P, Campo R, et al. Diagnosis of endometriosis: pelvic endoscopy and imaging techniques. Best Pract Res Clin Obstet Gynaecol 2004;18(2):285–303.
68. Abrao MS, Podgaec S, Dias JA, et al. Diagnosis of rectovaginal endometriosis. Hum Reprod 2008;23(10):2386 [author reply: 2386–7].
69. Goncalves MO, Podgaec S, Dias JA Jr, et al. Transvaginal ultrasonography with bowel preparation is able to predict the number of lesions and rectosigmoid layers affected in cases of deep endometriosis, defining surgical strategy. Hum Reprod 2010;25(3):665–71.
70. Reid S, Lu C, Casikar I, et al. Prediction of pouch of Douglas obliteration in women with suspected endometriosis using a new real-time dynamic transvaginal ultrasound technique: the sliding sign. Ultrasound Obstet Gynecol 2013;41(6):685–91.
71. Bazot M, Darai E, Hourani R, et al. Deep pelvic endometriosis: MR imaging for diagnosis and prediction of extension of disease. Radiology 2004;232(2):379–89.
72. Rossi L, Palazzo L, Yazbeck C, et al. Can rectal endoscopic sonography be used to predict infiltration depth in patients with deep infiltrating endometriosis of the rectum? Ultrasound Obstet Gynecol 2014;43(3):322–7.

73. Bazot M, Bornier C, Dubernard G, et al. Accuracy of magnetic resonance imaging and rectal endoscopic sonography for the prediction of location of deep pelvic endometriosis. Hum Reprod 2007;22(5):1457–63.
74. Khong SY, Bignardi T, Luscombe G, et al. Is pouch of Douglas obliteration a marker of bowel endometriosis? J Minim Invasive Gynecol 2011;18(3):333–7.
75. Remorgida V, Ferrero S, Fulcheri E, et al. Bowel endometriosis: presentation, diagnosis, and treatment. Obstet Gynecol Surv 2007;62(7):461–70.
76. Angioni S, Pontis A, Dessole M, et al. Pain control and quality of life after laparoscopic en-block resection of deep infiltrating endometriosis (DIE) vs. incomplete surgical treatment with or without GnRHa administration after surgery. Arch Gynecol Obstet 2014. http://dx.doi.org/10.1007/s00404-014-3411-5.
77. Chapron C, Vercellini P, Barakat H, et al. Management of ovarian endometriomas. Hum Reprod Update 2002;8(6):591–7.
78. Giudice LC. Clinical practice. Endometriosis. N Engl J Med 2010;362(25): 2389–98.
79. Raffi F, Metwally M, Amer S. The impact of excision of ovarian endometrioma on ovarian reserve: a systematic review and meta-analysis. J Clin Endocrinol Metab 2012;97(9):3146–54.
80. Alborzi S, Ravanbakhsh R, Parsanezhad ME, et al. A comparison of follicular response of ovaries to ovulation induction after laparoscopic ovarian cystectomy or fenestration and coagulation versus normal ovaries in patients with endometrioma. Fertil Steril 2007;88(2):507–9.
81. Hart RJ, Hickey M, Maouris P, et al. Excisional surgery versus ablative surgery for ovarian endometriomata. Cochrane Database Syst Rev 2008;(2):CD004992.
82. Muzii L, Panici PB. Combined technique of excision and ablation for the surgical treatment of ovarian endometriomas: the way forward? Reprod Biomed Online 2010;20(2):300–2.
83. Saito N, Okuda K, Yuguchi H, et al. Compared with cystectomy, is ovarian vaporization of endometriotic cysts truly more effective in maintaining ovarian reserve? J Minim Invasive Gynecol 2014;21(5):804–10.
84. Vercellini P, Aimi G, Busacca M, et al. Laparoscopic uterosacral ligament resection for dysmenorrhea associated with endometriosis: results of a randomized, controlled trial. Fertil Steril 2003;80(2):310–9.
85. Zullo F, Palomba S, Zupi E, et al. Long-term effectiveness of presacral neurectomy for the treatment of severe dysmenorrhea due to endometriosis. J Am Assoc Gynecol Laparosc 2004;11(1):23–8.
86. Matorras R, Elorriaga MA, Pijoan JI, et al. Recurrence of endometriosis in women with bilateral adnexectomy (with or without total hysterectomy) who received hormone replacement therapy. Fertil Steril 2002;77(2):303–8.
87. Practice Committee of the American Society for Reproductive Medicine. Endometriosis and infertility: a committee opinion. Fertil Steril 2012;98(3):591–8.
88. Jacobson TZ, Barlow DH, Koninckx PR, et al. Laparoscopic surgery for subfertility associated with endometriosis. Cochrane Database Syst Rev 2002;(4):CD001398.
89. Sallam HN, Garcia-Velasco JA, Dias S, et al. Long-term pituitary down-regulation before in vitro fertilization (IVF) for women with endometriosis. Cochrane Database Syst Rev 2006;(1):CD004635.
90. Hughes E, Brown J, Collins JJ, et al. Ovulation suppression for endometriosis. Cochrane Database Syst Rev 2007;(3):CD000155.
91. Deaton JL, Gibson M, Blackmer KM, et al. A randomized, controlled trial of clomiphene citrate and intrauterine insemination in couples with unexplained infertility or surgically corrected endometriosis. Fertil Steril 1990;54(6):1083–8.

92. Fedele L, Bianchi S, Marchini M, et al. Superovulation with human menopausal gonadotropins in the treatment of infertility associated with minimal or mild endometriosis: a controlled randomized study. Fertil Steril 1992;58(1):28–31.
93. Barnhart K, Dunsmoor-Su R, Coutifaris C. Effect of endometriosis on in vitro fertilization. Fertil Steril 2002;77(6):1148–55.
94. Stern JE, Brown MB, Wantman E, et al. Live birth rates and birth outcomes by diagnosis using linked cycles from the SART CORS database. J Assist Reprod Genet 2013;30(11):1445–50.
95. Werbrouck E, Spiessens C, Meuleman C, et al. No difference in cycle pregnancy rate and in cumulative live-birth rate between women with surgically treated minimal to mild endometriosis and women with unexplained infertility after controlled ovarian hyperstimulation and intrauterine insemination. Fertil Steril 2006;86(3): 566–71.

Abnormal Uterine Bleeding in Reproductive-aged Women

Michelle L. Matthews, MD

KEYWORDS

- Menorrhagia • Menstrual bleeding • Sonohysterography • Uterine bleeding
- Anovulation

KEY POINTS

- Abnormal uterine bleeding (AUB) is one of the most common gynecologic complaints in reproductive-aged women.
- The new International Federation of Gynecology and Obstetrics classification system should be used to classify all forms of AUB.
- Anovulatory bleeding is the most common nonanatomic cause of AUB and is most often observed in adolescents and perimenopausal patients as well as in some women with other pathologic conditions (eg, obesity, polycystic ovarian syndrome).
- Most AUB unrelated to uterine structural abnormalities is amenable to medical management, including hormonal treatments, antifibrinolyics, and nonsteroidal antiinflammatories.
- Uterine structural abnormalities that cause AUB (ie, polyps, fibroids, adenomyosis) generally require surgical management.

INTRODUCTION

Abnormal uterine bleeding (AUB) is one of the most common gynecologic conditions experienced by women of reproductive age. AUB is the cause of approximately one-third of all visits to gynecologists among premenopausal women and more than 70% of office visits among perimenopausal and postmenopausal women. The estimated annual direct cost of AUB in 2007 was approximately $1 billion, with indirect economic costs of $12 billion.[1] These figures do not account for intangible costs and productivity loss. Health care providers should be aware of the most common causes and treatment options for AUB given the high prevalence of the condition.

The term AUB has traditionally described all forms of abnormal vaginal bleeding. The use of other terms for vaginal bleeding, such as dysfunctional uterine bleeding,

The author has nothing to disclose.
Reproductive Endocrinology, Carolinas HealthCare System, 1025 Morehead Medical Drive, Suite 500, Charlotte, NC 28204, USA
E-mail address: michelle.matthews@carolinashealthcare.org

Obstet Gynecol Clin N Am 42 (2015) 103–115
http://dx.doi.org/10.1016/j.ogc.2014.09.006
0889-8545/15/$ – see front matter © 2015 Elsevier Inc. All rights reserved.

obgyn.theclinics.com

polymenorrhea, menorrhagia, metrorrhagia, and hypermenorrhea, has caused confusion for many health care providers. In addition, the terminology used in other countries for the various gynecologic causes of vaginal bleeding has not been congruent with the medical definitions used in the United States. In response to these concerns, the International Federation of Gynecology and Obstetrics (FIGO) published a new nomenclature system in 2011 to create an internationally accepted classification system.[2] This system allows for consistent terminology in describing AUB and facilitates communication between health care providers, and also provides a format to accurately analyze effective medical and surgical treatments. The system classifies AUB by bleeding pattern as well as cause and includes 9 main categories. The system was recently accepted by the American College of Obstetricians and Gynecologists (ACOG) and an update to the AUB 2000 practice bulletin was published in 2013.[3] This article reviews the FIGO classification system as well as evaluation and management options.

NORMAL VERSUS ABNORMAL UTERINE BLEEDING
Normal Menstrual Bleeding

Most ovulatory menstrual cycles last between 21 and 35 days. The duration of normal menstrual flow is generally 5 days, with most blood loss occurring within the first 3 days.[4] The average amount of bleeding during the menstrual cycle is 30 to 40 mL. Only 10% of women have more than 80 mL, which is considered abnormal. Approximately 65% of patients have anemia when menstrual blood loss exceeds 80 mL per month.[5] Approximately 25% of patients with measured blood loss of less than 60 mL consider their menstrual cycles to be heavy. Therefore, research supports that it is difficult for most women to accurately estimate menstrual blood loss and differentiate between normal and heavy menstrual bleeding.

Menstrual cycles are predictable in most women, but the length of the cycle can vary by a few days each month and is more unpredictable during puberty and perimenopause. The menstrual cycle comprises the follicular phase and the luteal phase. These phases are controlled through complex interactions between the ovary, hypothalamus, pituitary gland, and uterus. The follicular phase is initiated by recruitment of an oocyte in response to ovarian stimulation from the pituitary. The follicular phase is marked by estrogen dominance, and is typically of a variable length secondary to hormonal fluctuations during oocyte selection and maturation. These fluctuations are most prominent during the pubertal and perimenopausal transitions.

The luteal phase is marked by progesterone dominance after ovulation and is generally a more fixed length of 12 to 14 days. Menstruation occurs as estrogen and progesterone levels decline at the end of the luteal phase if pregnancy does not occur. Dysfunction at the level of the hypothalamus, pituitary, or ovary can interfere with ovulation and prevent routine shedding of the endometrium, which may result in heavy menstrual bleeding, intermenstrual spotting/bleeding, or both.

Abnormal Uterine Bleeding

AUB has been defined by FIGO as bleeding from the uterine corpus that is abnormal in regularity, volume, frequency, or duration and occurs in the absence of pregnancy.[2] The causes of AUB are classified as "related to uterine structural abnormalities" and "unrelated to uterine structural abnormalities." AUB is classified by one or more letters that indicate the cause. These are categorized by the acronym PALM-COEIN (polyp, adenomyosis, leiomyoma, malignancy, and hyperplasia; coagulopathy, ovulatory dysfunction, endometrial, iatrogenic, and not otherwise classified). In addition, patterns of AUB are described as either heavy menstrual bleeding (previously referred to as menorrhagia), or intermenstrual bleeding (instead of metrorrhagia). Leiomyomas may be subclassified as either submucosal or those that do not affect the uterine cavity (**Fig. 1**). Abnormal bleeding associated with the use of exogenous steroids (ie, hormonal treatments), intrauterine systems (IUSs) or devices, or other systemic or local agents are classified as iatrogenic, whereas the remainder of rare or ill-defined causes are categorized as not yet classified.

AUB may be acute or chronic. Acute AUB refers to an episode of heavy bleeding that is of sufficient quantity to require immediate intervention to prevent further blood loss. The amount of bleeding may be subjectively excessive as determined by the health care provider and/or associated with other signs of significant blood loss, such as hemodynamic instability or anemia. Patients should be assessed to determine the level of acuity and the most likely cause of the bleeding to tailor appropriate treatment.[6] Acute AUB may be an isolated event or occur in a background of chronic AUB. The evaluation of acute AUB is similar to evaluation of chronic AUB after assessment of hemodynamic status and assuring stability of the patient. Although this article focuses primarily on chronic AUB, medical treatments for acute AUB are discussed.

EVALUATION
History and Physical Examination

It is important to have an organized and evidence-based approach to evaluation and management of AUB. The evaluation of women with AUB includes a thorough medical history and physical examination, appropriate laboratory and imaging tests, and

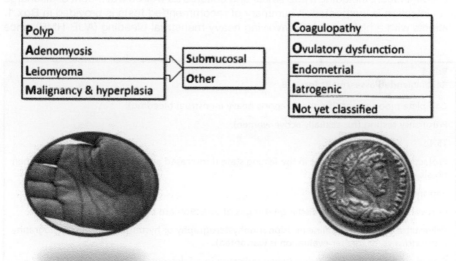

Fig. 1. Basic classification system. The leiomyoma category (L) is subdivided into patients with at least 1 submucosal myoma (L_{sm}) and those with myomas that do not affect the endometrial cavity (L_0). (*From* Munro MG, Critchley HO, Broder MS, et al. FIGO Working Group on Menstrual Disorders. FIGO classification system (PALM-COEIN) for causes of abnormal uterine bleeding in nongravid women of reproductive age. Int J Gynaecol Obstet 2011;113:5; with permission.)

consideration of age-related factors that may help to focus the differential diagnosis. The medical history should include a patient description of her bleeding patterns as well as any recent changes in amount, duration, frequency, and associated pain. The history should also include questions about other bleeding problems (eg, epistaxis, bleeding gums, frequent bruising), particularly in adolescents presenting with acute bleeding and adults with chronic heavy menstrual bleeding and anemia. Pertinent medical conditions should also be elicited (eg, thyroid disease, hypertension, renal disease, anorexia/bulimia, psychiatric conditions, and other chronic medical conditions) because these may contribute to ovulatory dysfunction. Any pertinent family history should be discussed (ie, bleeding disorders/coagulopathies) as well as other gynecologic and obstetric history. A list of medications should also be obtained because some may contribute to AUB (ie, hormones, anticoagulants/fibrinolytics, psychotropics).

The physical examination may also reveal findings that contribute to AUB. Any signs of thyroid disease (nodule, goiter), hyperprolactinemia (galactorrhea), polycystic ovarian syndrome (PCOS) (acne, hirsutism), should be documented. Signs of a bleeding disorder may include petechiae, epistaxis, and ecchymoses. A pelvic examination, including a speculum and bimanual examination, should evaluate for any signs of trauma, external or internal vaginal/cervical lesions, infection, and uterine enlargement.

Laboratory Testing

Laboratory testing depends on the patient history and physical examination. Initial evaluation may include a complete blood count (CBC), thyroid-stimulating hormone (TSH), prolactin, and pregnancy test. Other testing may be indicated based on the pelvic examination, including a pap smear and cultures as well as wet mount of discharge if an infection is suspected. A summary of recommended tests is provided in **Box 1**. Patients with a history of AUB involving heavy menstrual bleeding (AUB-HMB) since

---

Box 1
Recommended assessment for AUB

Complete blood count (if patient reports heavy menstrual bleeding).

Pregnancy testing (for sexually active women).

TSH.

Prolactin level testing (repeat in the fasting state if increased and in the follicular phase when possible).

Pap smear if indicated.

Cervical cultures (if vaginal discharge or signs of infection are present).

Pelvic ultrasonography (saline infusion sonohysterography or hysteroscopy if ultrasonography is inconclusive or further evaluation is warranted).

Screening for bleeding disorders (when indicated in adolescents with heavy menstrual bleeding or adults with chronic menstrual bleeding and a positive screening history).

Endometrial biopsy in women more than 45 years old. Obtain if younger than 45 years if patient has risk factors for endometrial hyperplasia or malignancy.

Data from American College of Obstetricians and Gynecologists. Practice bulletin no. 128: diagnosis of abnormal uterine bleeding in reproductive-aged women. Obstet Gynecol 2012;120:197–206.

menarche or with either postpartum hemorrhage or surgery-related bleeding, including dental procedures, should be screened for bleeding disorders. Other indications for bleeding disorder testing include frequent bleeding from the gums, epistaxis or easy bruising (1 or more times per month), or a family history of a bleeding disorder. Initial evaluation should include a CBC and platelets, prothrombin time, partial thromboplastin time, fibrinogen, or thrombin time (optional). If these tests are abnormal the patient should be evaluated more thoroughly for an underlying bleeding disorder such as von Willebrand disease, which is the most common of the inherited bleeding disorders in women.[7]

Uterine Evaluation

Uterine evaluation for AUB should include imaging studies and an endometrial biopsy when indicated. The risk of endometrial cancer is 6.2% in women aged 35 to 44 years but increases more significantly to 13.6 to 24 per 1 million woman-years for women aged 40 to 50 years. Endometrial biopsy should be performed as a first-line test in patients more than 45 years of age. An endometrial biopsy should also be obtained in patients younger than 45 years with a history of exposure to unopposed estrogen (ie, PCOS, obesity), those who fail medical management and have persistent AUB, or those who have any irregularity in the appearance of the endometrium on ultrasonography.[8] Endometrial biopsies are most often performed with a endometrial suction device, which has a sensitivity of 81% and specificity of more than 98% as long as a sufficient sample is obtained.[9] However, this is a blinded procedure and may miss small lesions. Therefore, patients with a normal endometrial biopsy (ie, no hyperplasia or cancer) should have additional endometrial assessment with ultrasonography if not already performed, as well as possible dilation and curettage and hysteroscopy if symptoms persist.

Evaluation of the uterus for anatomic causes of bleeding should include imaging studies. Visualization of the uterine architecture with either transabdominal or transvaginal ultrasonography is a valuable tool to assess anatomic causes of bleeding. Transvaginal ultrasonography generally provides better visualization of the uterus and ovaries; however, it may not be the preferred method for patients uncomfortable with the vaginal probe. A full bladder improves visualization of the uterus during transabdominal ultrasonography. Ultrasonography may reveal either endometrial or myometrial abnormalities. Myometrial abnormalities most commonly include uterine leiomyomas or adenomyosis. Uterine leiomyomas (fibroids) are overgrowths of smooth muscle cells and are generally visualized as homogeneous, well-circumscribed lesions. Adenomyosis results from invagination of endometrial tissue into the myometrium and is typically more diffuse in appearance than leiomyomas. It is generally visualized on ultrasonography as a heterogeneous-appearing area with small cystic areas.

Ultrasonography ideally should be scheduled between days 4 and 6 of the menstrual cycle, when the endometrium is the thinnest. Endometrial thickness varies during the menstrual cycle. It is typically 4 to 8 mm during the follicular phase, and 8 to 14 mm during the luteal phase.[10] Ultrasonography performed during the follicular phase may be more likely to detect subtle abnormalities within the endometrium, such as small polyps or intracavitary fibroids. The size and location of all abnormalities should be noted. Further evaluation is warranted by either saline infusion sonohysterography or hysteroscopy if an endometrial or intracavitary abnormality is suspected.

Saline infusion sonohysterography can determine the presence or absence of intracavitary lesions and the depth of myometrial involvement with leiomyomas. Saline infusion sonohysterography is an office-based imaging procedure that infuses saline into the endometrial cavity during transvaginal ultrasonography. The saline distends the uterine cavity to enhance the visualization of intracavitary polyps and myomas, which may otherwise be obscured by adjacent endometrial tissue (**Fig. 2**).

Saline infusion sonohysterography has a high sensitivity (96%–100%) and a high negative predictive value (94%–100%) in evaluating the uterus and endometrium for disorders.[11,12] Saline infusion sonohysterography should be performed in the follicular phase of the cycle after menstruation has ended but before ovulation to ensure that the patient is not pregnant and to optimize image quality. Saline infusion sonography has similar diagnostic accuracy to office hysteroscopy (81.3% vs 87.5%, respectively) but is generally less painful.[13]

Hysteroscopy is a technique that allows direct visualization of the uterine cavity by placing a thin telescopic instrument through the cervix into the uterus. It permits full visualization of the endometrial cavity and endocervix and may be performed either in an operating room or office setting. It is helpful in diagnosing and treating focal or diffuse lesions. It may be performed diagnostically instead of saline infusion sonography, or operatively to confirm and treat any visualized abnormality. Hysteroscopy can assist in the diagnosis of atrophy, endometrial polyps, leiomyomas, and other endometrial abnormalities. Tissue samples may be sent for pathologic evaluation to confirm the diagnosis and rule out endometrial hyperplasia and cancer. An algorithm for uterine evaluation is provided in **Fig. 3**.

MANAGEMENT (SURGICAL AND NONSURGICAL)
Medical Management

The goals of medical management for patients with AUB are regulation of menstrual cycles for patients with AUB involving intermenstrual bleeding (AUB-IMB), and decreased menstrual blood loss for patients with AUB-HMB. Medications to reduce menstrual blood loss include hormonal treatments, antifibrinolyics, and prostaglandin synthetase inhibitors. The choice of treatment depends on its appropriateness considering other medical conditions and the preference of, and tolerability by, the patient. A summary of medical treatment options is provided in **Box 2**.

Medical management is preferred to surgical treatment of most patients unless an anatomic cause for bleeding is identified (ie, polyp, fibroid, hyperplasia, cancer). Medical management with hormones is often recommended for patients with AUB not related to an anatomic cause because the cause in these patients is often anovulation. Correction of the underlying hormonal imbalance for patients with anovulation frequently results in improvement in AUB-HMB and AUB-IMB.

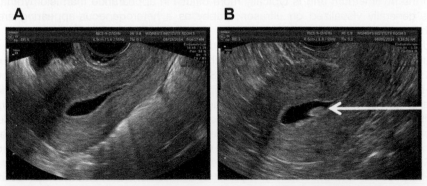

Fig. 2. Sonohysterography. (*A*) Normal intrauterine cavity. (*B*) Uterine filling defect (*arrow*).

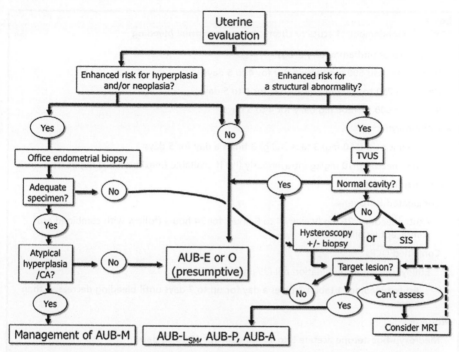

Fig. 3. Uterine evaluation of AUB. AUB-A, abnormal uterine bleeding-adenomyosis; AUB-E, abnormal uterine bleeding-endometrial or AUB-O, abnormal uterine bleeding-ovulatory dysfunction; AUB-L$_{SM}$, abnormal uterine bleeding-submucosal leiomyoma; AUB-M, abnormal uterine bleeding-malignancy or hyperplasia; AUB-P, abnormal uterine bleeding-polyp; CA, carcinoma; SIS, saline instilled sonography; TVUS, transvaginal ultrasonography. (*From* Munro MG, Critchley HO, Broder MS, et al. FIGO Working Group on Menstrual Disorders. FIGO classification system (PALM-COEIN) for causes of abnormal uterine bleeding in nongravid women of reproductive age. Int J Gynaecol Obstet 2011;113:3–13; with permission.)

Hormonal therapies

Hormonal treatments for AUB include estrogens or progestins, given either independently or in combination (ie, combined oral contraceptive pills [OCPs]). The goal of hormonal therapy is to restore the sequence of synchronized growth of the endometrium with estrogen and stabilization with progesterone before endometrial shedding at menstruation. Estrogens stimulate endometrial tissue growth over the surface of the denuded endometrium to stop menstrual bleeding. There is also evidence that estrogens stimulate clotting at the capillary level, which contributes to cessation of menstruation.[14] Most forms of hormonal treatment are effective for both acute and chronic bleeding but the dosing is adjusted according to the acuity of the bleeding. In addition, most forms of hormonal treatment are approved for contraceptive indications, but are often used for medical management of AUB.

Estrogens are the most effective hormonal treatment of acute bleeding. Intravenous conjugated equine estrogens stop bleeding in 70% of patients within 4 to 8 hours compared with 30% with placebo.[15] Bleeding also stops for almost 90% of patients with acute bleeding by administration of combined OCPs 3 times daily for 1 week.[16] Only intravenous conjugated equine estrogen is approved for treatment of acute AUB requiring hospitalization, although other routes and doses of administration of estrogens may be effective. Estrogen therapy should be continued for at least 3 weeks

---

Box 2
Medical management of acute or chronic heavy menstrual bleeding

Nonsteroidal antiinflammatory drugs

  Mefenamic acid 500 mg twice a day for 4 to 5 days

  Naproxen 250 to 500 mg twice a day for 4 to 5 days

  Ibuprofen 600 to 1200 mg daily for 4 to 5 days

Antifibrinolytics[a]

  Tranexamic acid (650 mg) 3 tabs (1.3 g) 3 times a day for 5 days

    Acute bleeding: 10 mg/kg intravenously (IV) if available (maximum 600 mg/dose)

Hormonal treatments

  Conjugated estrogens

    Acute bleeding: 25 mg IV every 4 to 6 hours for 24 hours (follow with combined oral contraceptive pills [OCPs])

  Combined OCPs

    Ethinyl estradiol combination pill (35 μg)[b]

      Acute bleeding: 1 tablet 3 times a day for up to 7 days until bleeding decreases, then taper

Progestins

  Medroxyprogesterone acetate 5 to 10 mg daily for 12 to 14 days[a]

    Acute bleeding: 10 mg every 4 hours (up to 80 mg/d for acute bleeding) then every 6 hours for 4 days, then every 8 hours for 3 days, then every 12 hours for 2 days to 2 weeks, then daily

  Norethindrone 5 mg daily for 5–10 days[a]

    Acute bleeding: 5 to 10 mg every 4 hours until bleeding stops, then every 6 hours for 4 days, then every 8 hours for 3 days, then every 12 hours for 2 days to 2 weeks, then daily

  Levonorgestrel intrauterine system (approved for use for 5 years)

[a]*Data from* James AH, Kouides PA, Abdul-Kadir R, et al. Evaluation and management of acute menorrhagia in women with and without underlying bleeding disorders: consensus from an international expert panel. Eur J Obstet Gynecol Reprod Biol 2011;158:124–34.
[b]*Data from* American College of Obstetricians and Gynecologists. ACOG committee opinion no. 557: management of acute abnormal uterine bleeding in nonpregnant reproductive-aged women. Obstet Gynecol 2013;121(4):891–6.

---

to prevent immediate subsequent bleeding episodes. Care should be taken when prescribing higher dose estrogen therapy for extended periods because of a possible increased risk of thromboembolic events. Standard doses of estrogens are typically sufficient to control bleeding once the acute bleeding event has been treated. Estrogen therapy should be followed by a progestin for 10 days each month to schedule a synchronized withdrawal bleed. A scheduled program of an estrogen followed by progestin should be continued monthly for most patients to regulate further AUB.

There are several progestin-only treatments, including medroxyprogesterone acetate, megestrol acetate, norethindrone acetate, depomedroxyprogesterone acetate, the etonogestrel implant, and the levonorgestrel IUS (ie, intrauterine system). Progestins induce secretory changes in an estrogen-primed endometrium. Therefore, it is important to remember that progestins do not provide benefit to women with bleeding secondary to low estrogen levels with a thin endometrium on ultrasonography. They are most likely to be effective in patients with anovulatory bleeding and adequate estrogen (ie, PCOS). Contraindications include known or suspected pregnancy, undiagnosed vaginal bleeding, known or suspected breast cancer, active deep vein thrombosis, pulmonary embolism, or history of these conditions; active or recent stroke or myocardial infarction; and impaired liver function. Side effects are generally nausea, weight gain and fluid retention, mood changes, edema, as well as irregular bleeding.

Progestins may be given continuously or cyclically. Cyclic progestin therapy once per month for 10 to 14 days allows for a synchronized withdrawal bleed. Progestins antagonize estrogen and are effective to stop endometrial growth during the luteal phase. This treatment prevents excessive amounts of endometrium from developing during each menstrual cycle. Progestins cause endometrial atrophy when given continuously and are used effectively in higher dosages for patients with endometrial hyperplasia. Oral progestins given in a cyclic fashion do not prevent ovulation. Patients should be advised to use alternate forms of contraception if they are not actively trying to conceive.

There are no studies comparing progestins with placebo for treatment of heavy menstrual bleeding. A review of published studies reported that oral progestins offered no advantage compared with nonhormonal treatment with tranexamic acid or nonsteroidal antiinflammatory drugs (NSAIDs). However, there was a benefit of the levonorgestrel IUS compared with oral progestins for women with ovulatory cycles. The levonorgestrel IUS was also better tolerated than oral progestin.[17] This effect is likely secondary to its local effect on the endometrium without the systemic side effects of oral administration. Although effective for treating heavy menstrual bleeding, approximately 36% of patients have the IUS removed at 2 years because of lack of effectiveness.[18] Advantages of the levonorgestrel IUS include its efficacy for contraception and that it may remain in place for 5 years. However, the levonorgestrel IUS is not cost-effective for short-term use.

Combined hormonal contraceptives are available in oral, patch, and vaginal ring forms. Combined hormonal contraceptives work well for most patients with bleeding because they contain both the estrogen and progestin agents. They are also well suited for patients requesting contraception or who are not actively trying to conceive. Highly significant reductions in menstrual blood loss have been reported with oral contraceptives (43%); however, there have been no well-designed placebo-controlled trials.[19] There have not been any large trials evaluating the oral route compared with other routes of administration of combined hormonal contraception. However, all routes should be similarly effective for control of heavy menstrual bleeding.

There are many other advantages of combined oral contraceptives for certain patient populations. Perimenopausal patients may note improvement in hot flashes as well as other menopausal symptoms related to low estrogen levels. Adolescents may experience improvement of acne. Patients with polycystic ovarian syndrome may have decreases in acne and hirsutism, and have a decreased risk of endometrial cancer. Combined hormonal contraceptives can increase levels of factor VIII and von Willebrand factor, which may benefit patients with underlying coagulopathies.

Nonsteroidal antiinflammatory drugs
Nonsteroidal antiinflammatories are a category of medications that reduce prostaglandin levels by inhibiting the enzyme cyclooxygenase. Several NSAIDs have been evaluated for patients with AUB-HMB, including mefenamic acid (MFA), naproxen,

ibuprofen, meclofenamic acid, diclofenac, indomethacin, and acetylsalicylic acid. However, the most commonly used are MFA, naproxen, and ibuprofen. The endometrium of women with heavy menstrual bleeding has been shown to have higher levels of the prostaglandins E2 and F2α and inhibition of prostaglandin is the presumed mechanism for reduced blood loss.[20] They are contraindicated in patients with platelet disorders or on anticoagulants. They are generally not recommended for people with kidney disease, heart failure, or cirrhosis, or for people who take diuretics. The most common side effect is gastrointestinal upset.

Menstrual blood loss is reduced with NSAIDs by up to 35% for about 75% of patients with heavy menstrual bleeding.[21] There are also limited data directly comparing OCPs with NSAIDs. A large meta-analysis of NSAIDs compared with other medical management for control of menstrual blood loss found that NSAIDs are effective but that tranexamic acid or the levonorgestrel IUS are more effective. The data comparing the effectiveness of different NSAIDs are limited, but suggest that there is no significant difference between MFA and naproxen. However, side effects may be less common with MFA.[22]

Antifibrinolytics

Plasminogen activators have been found at higher than expected concentrations in the endometrium of women with heavy menstrual bleeding.[23] Plasminogen activators are enzymes that result in fibrinolysis and degradation of blood clots. Plasminogen activator inhibitors decrease fibrinolysis and promote clot formation, which decreases menstrual blood loss. Tranexamic acid is an antifibrinolyic therapy approved for medical treatment of menorrhagia. It reversibly binds to lysine binding sites on plasminogen molecules. It is associated with a significant reduction in mean blood loss (40%–50%) in women with heavy menstrual bleeding compared with placebo. It was found to be more effective that oral progestin or MFA.[24] Tranexamic acid may be prescribed to decrease menstrual blood loss for patients with bleeding disorders such as von Willebrand disease, but is not approved for use in patients less than 18 years of age. It is available over the counter in many countries, but requires a prescription in the United States. It is generally well tolerated with few side effects. The most common side effects reported are nausea and dizziness. It is contraindicated in patients with active thromboembolic disease, disseminated intravascular coagulation, macroscopic hematuria, and color blindness. It should be used with caution with patients at risk of clotting; however, long-term use has not been associated with a higher risk of thrombosis compared with the risk of spontaneous thrombosis in untreated women.[25]

Surgical Treatment

Surgical treatment of AUB may also be considered for patients who do not improve with medical management or have anatomic causes for bleeding. Several surgical options exist. However, definitive treatment with hysterectomy should only be considered for patients who have completed childbearing or have contraindications from, or are unresponsive to, medical management. Surgery is generally recommended for patients with anatomic causes of bleeding, whereas medical management is the mainstay of treatment of nonanatomic causes. However, approximately 80% of patients with heavy menstrual bleeding treated with surgery have no anatomic disorder.[26]

Surgical treatment of fibroids typically includes myomectomy (removal of fibroids) by hysteroscopy, laparoscopy, or laparotomy. Other nonmedical treatments for fibroids include embolization, cryomyolysis, and magnetic resonance–guided focal ultrasonography ablation. Embolization is generally not recommended for patients who are still interested in childbearing because it may decrease uterine and subsequent placental blood flow. There are also limited pregnancy outcome data on other treatments besides myomectomy for patients interested in fertility. Surgical treatment of polyps is typically hysteroscopic resection. Adenomyosis is often difficult to treat surgically because of its diffuse growth into the myometrium. However, it may be resected in a similar fashion to a myomectomy, although the borders are most difficult to identify. Surgical treatments for AUB in patients who have completed childbearing include endometrial resection/ablation and hysterectomy.

Endometrial ablation techniques were developed in the 1980s. The first method was hysteroscopic ablation with laser photovaporization.[27] Subsequent techniques involved either ablating the endometrium with a rollerball, or resecting it with a cautery loop under direct observation with hysteroscopy. The newer second-generation techniques for ablation use either microwave energy, thermal balloon, radiofrequency, cryotherapy, or heated water. The second-generation modalities are quicker, some may be performed in the office, are generally less expensive, and do not require hysteroscopy. They seem to have similar results for treatment of heavy menstrual bleeding, with similar patient satisfaction.[28]

Endometrial ablation is often preferred by patients compared with definitive surgical hysterectomy because of quicker return to normal function and avoidance of major surgery. Vaginal discharge is the most commonly reported side effect as the endometrium undergoes necrosis. Patients having endometrial ablation generally experience immediate decreases in bleeding; however, many patients need subsequent hysterectomy. The probability of a woman requiring a repeat procedure is higher than with a definitive hysterectomy. The relative risk at 1 year is 14.9 (95% confidence interval [CI], 5.2–42.6) and increases to 36.4 (95% CI, 5.1–259.2) at 4 years.[29]

Definitive surgical treatment of AUB is hysterectomy. Approximately 600,000 hysterectomies are performed annually in the United States, and approximately 20 million American women have had a hysterectomy.[30] Hysterectomy is efficacious for the management of AUB because it removes the source of bleeding. It treats bleeding from both anatomic and nonanatomic causes. However, a hysterectomy has risks, including urinary incontinence, sexual dysfunction, and other signs of estrogen deprivation if the ovaries also removed. Other immediate risks include infection, bleeding, and mortality of 1 to 6 per 1000 women when performed for benign causes.[31]

SUMMARY/DISCUSSION

AUB is a common problem in reproductive-aged women and has many causes. There is a new international classification system developed by FIGO that has been supported by ACOG. Health care providers should have an evidence-based approach to evaluation and management. Medical management is effective to control most AUB related to nonanatomic causes. Medical management may include hormonal and/or nonhormonal treatments and should be tailored to the patient depending on side effect profiles and contraindications. Hormonal therapies decrease bleeding for most patients. Nonhormonal treatments such as NSAIDs and antifibrinolytics are also effective and may be used in conjunction with or instead of hormonal treatments. Patients with anatomic causes for bleeding may benefit from medical management, but may require surgical treatment of the underlying abnormality (ie, polyp, myomas, adenomyosis). Surgical treatment of patients who have completed childbearing may include endometrial ablation or hysterectomy.

REFERENCES

1. Liu Z, Doan QV, Blumenthal P, et al. A systematic review evaluating health-related quality of life, work impairment and healthcare costs and utilization in abnormal uterine bleeding. Value Health 2007;10(8):183–94.
2. Munro MG, Critchley HO, Broder MS, et al, FIGO Working Group on Menstrual Disorders. FIGO classification system (PALM-COEIN) for causes of abnormal uterine bleeding in nongravid women of reproductive age. Int J Gynaecol Obstet 2011;113:3–13.
3. American College of Obstetricians and Gynecologists. ACOG committee opinion no. 136: management of abnormal uterine bleeding associated with ovulatory dysfunction. Obstet Gynecol 2013;122(1):176–85.
4. American College of Obstetricians and Gynecologists. ACOG committee opinion no. 349: menstruation in girls and adolescents: using the menstrual cycle as a vital sign. Obstet Gynecol 2006;108:1323–8.
5. Hallberg L, Hogdahl AM, Nilson L, et al. Menstrual blood loss–a population study. Acta Obstet Gynecol Scand 1966;45:320–51.
6. American College of Obstetricians and Gynecologists. ACOG committee opinion no. 557: management of acute abnormal uterine bleeding in nonpregnant reproductive-aged women. Obstet Gynecol 2013;121(4):891–6.
7. Von Willebrand disease evaluation and management. Available at: https://www.nhlbi.nih.gov/health-pro/guidelines/current/von-willebrand-guidelines/full-report/3-diagnosis-evaluation.htm. Accessed September 1, 2014.
8. Haidopoulos D, Simou M, Akrivos N, et al. Risk factors in women 40 years of age and younger with endometrial cancer. Acta Obstet Gynecol Scand 2010;89:1326–30.
9. Dijkhuizen FP, Mol BW, Brölmann HA, et al. The accuracy of endometrial sampling in the diagnosis of patients with endometrial carcinoma and hyperplasia: a meta-analysis. Cancer 2000;89(8):1765.
10. Goldstein SR, Zeltser I, Horan CK, et al. Ultrasonography-based triage for peri-menopausal patients with abnormal uterine bleeding. Am J Obstet Gynecol 1997;177:102–8.
11. Mihm LM, Quick VA, Brumfield JA, et al. The accuracy of endometrial biopsy and saline sonohysterography in the determination of the cause of abnormal uterine bleeding. Am J Obstet Gynecol 2002;186:858–60.
12. Williams CD, Marshburn PB. A prospective study of trans-vaginal hydrosonography in the evaluation of abnormal uterine bleeding. Am J Obstet Gynecol 1998;179:292–8.
13. Kelekci S, Kaya E, Alan M, et al. Comparison of transvaginal sonography infusion sonography, and office hysteroscopy in reproductive-aged women with or without abnormal uterine bleeding. Fertil Steril 2005;84(3):682–6.
14. Heistinger M, Stockenbuber F, Schneider B, et al. Effect of conjugated estrogens on platelet function and prostacyclin generation in CRF. Kidney Int 1990;38:1181–6.
15. Devore GR, Owen O, Kase N. Use of IV Premarin in the treatment of dysfunctional uterine bleeding–a double blind randomized controlled study. Obstet Gynecol 1982;59:285–91.
16. Munro MG, Mainor N, Basu R, et al. Oral medroxyprogesterone acetate and combination oral contraceptives for acute uterine bleeding: a randomized controlled trial. Obstet Gynecol 2006;108:924–9.
17. Lethaby A, Irvine G, Cameron IT. Cyclic progestogens for heavy menstrual bleeding (Review). Cochrane Database Syst Rev 2008;(1):CD001016. [meta-analyses].

18. Gupta J, Kai J, Middleton L, et al, ECLIPSE Trial Collaborative Group. Levonorgestrel intrauterine system versus medical therapy for menorrhea. N Engl J Med 2013;268:128–37.
19. Farquhar C, Brown J. Oral contraceptive pill for heavy menstrual bleeding (Review). Cochrane Database Syst Rev 2009;(4):CD000154. [meta-analyses].
20. Willman EA, Collins WD, Clayton SC. Studies on the involvement of prostaglandins in uterine symptomatology and pathology. Br J Obstet Gynaecol 1976;83:337–41.
21. Roy SN, Bhattacharya S. Benefits and risks of pharmacological agents used for the treatment of menorrhagia. Drug Saf 2004;27(2):75–90.
22. Lethaby A, Duckitt K, Farquhar C. Non-steroidal anti-inflammatory drugs for heavy menstrual bleeding (Review). Cochrane Database Syst Rev 2007;(4):CD000400. [meta-analyses].
23. Gleeson NC. Cyclic changes in endometrial tissue plasminogen activator and plasminogen activator inhibitor type 1 in women with normal menstruation and essential menorrhagia. Am J Obstet Gynecol 1994;171(1):178–83.
24. Lethaby A, Farquhar C, Cooke I. Antifibrinolytics for heavy menstrual bleeding (Review). Cochrane Database Syst Rev 2000;(4):CD000249. [meta-analyses].
25. Ryobi G. Tranexamic acid effective treatment in heavy menstrual bleeding: clinical update on safety. Ther Adv 1991;4:1–8.
26. Clarke A, Black N, Rowe P, et al. Indications for and outcomes of total abdominal hysterectomy for benign disease: a prospective cohort study. Br J Obstet Gynaecol 1995;102:611–20.
27. Goldrath MH, Fuller TA, Segal S. Laser photovaporization of endometrium for the treatment of menorrhagia. Am J Obstet Gynecol 1981;140:14–9.
28. Lethaby A, Penninx J, Hicket M, et al. Endometrial resection and ablation techniques for heavy menstrual bleeding editorial group: Cochrane Menstrual Disorders and Subfertility Group. Cochrane Database Syst Rev 2013;(8):CD001501. [meta-analyses].
29. Fergusson RJ, Lethaby A, Shepperd S, et al. Endometrial resection and ablation versus hysterectomy for heavy menstrual bleeding. Cochrane Database Syst Rev 2013;(11):CD000329. [meta-analyses].
30. Centers for Disease Control and Prevention Online. Hysterectomy surveillance United States, 1994, 1999, 2002. Available at: http://www.cdc.gov/mmwr/preview/mmwrhtml/ss5105a1.htm. Accessed September 1, 2014.
31. McPherson K, Metcalfe MA, Herbert A, et al. Severe complications of hysterectomy: the VALUE study. BJOG 2004;111(7):688–94.

Recurrent Pregnancy Loss
Evaluation and Treatment

Lora Shahine, MD[a,b], Ruth Lathi, MD[c],*

KEYWORDS

- Recurrent pregnancy loss • Recurrent miscarriage • Recurrent fetal loss
- Recurrent embryonic loss

KEY POINTS

- Evaluation for women with recurrent pregnancy loss includes checking for uterine anomalies and parental chromosomal rearrangements and testing for antiphospholipid antibodies.
- Fifty percent of patients will have no definite cause for recurrent pregnancy loss after a thorough evaluation.
- The prognosis for a live birth in women with unexplained recurrent pregnancy loss is 50% to 80% without intervention with evidence-based treatments and supportive care.
- More than half of first-trimester miscarriages tested will have sporadic numeric chromosomal abnormalities.
- Chromosomal screening of embryos after in vitro fertilization has been proposed as a treatment option to reduced aneuploidy conceptions, but it has not been evaluated in randomized controlled studies.

BACKGROUND AND DEFINITIONS

The definitions of miscarriage and recurrent pregnancy loss (RPL) are important to review because they vary within the literature and clinical teaching. Classically, RPL is defined as 3 pregnancy losses before the twentieth week of gestation and excludes ectopic, molar, and biochemical pregnancies. The American Society of Reproductive Medicine (ASRM) states that, for the purposes of determining whether an evaluation for RPL is appropriate, pregnancy is defined as a clinical pregnancy documented by ultrasonography or histopathologic examination and that a clinical evaluation may proceed following 2 first-trimester pregnancy losses.[1] ASRM

The authors have nothing to disclose.
[a] Pacific NW Fertility and IVF Specialists, Seattle, WA, USA; [b] Division of Reproductive Endocrinology and Infertility, Department of Obstetrics and Gynecology, University of Washington School of Medicine, Seattle, WA, USA; [c] Division of Reproductive Endocrinology and Infertility, Stanford University School of Medicine, Stanford, CA, USA
* Corresponding author.
E-mail address: rlathi@stanford.edu

Obstet Gynecol Clin N Am 42 (2015) 117–134
http://dx.doi.org/10.1016/j.ogc.2014.10.002
0889-8545/15/$ – see front matter © 2015 Elsevier Inc. All rights reserved.

maintains that a threshold of 3 or more pregnancy losses should be used for epidemiologic studies.[1]

RPL may be considered a primary or secondary condition. Primary RPL refers to multiple pregnancy losses in which a patient has never had a live birth, and secondary RPL refers to multiple pregnancy losses in a patient who has had a live birth previously.[2] Definitions are provided in **Table 1**.

INCIDENCE

Clinically recognized pregnancy loss occurs in approximately 15% to 25% of all pregnancies.[1] If preclinical losses are included, pregnancy loss is estimated to be as high as 57%.[3–5] It is estimated that less than 5% of women will experience 2 consecutive pregnancy losses and that only 1% of women will experience 3 or more.[3] The incidence of miscarriage increases with age of the woman such that women less than 35 years old have a 9% to 12% risk of spontaneous loss in the first trimester,[4,5] but this risk increases to 50% in women aged 40 years and older.[5–7]

EVALUATION AND TREATMENT BY CAUSE

RPL has been associated with factors related to genetics, age, antiphospholipid syndrome, uterine anomalies, thrombophilias, hormonal or metabolic disorders, infection, autoimmunity, sperm parameters, and lifestyle issues. With a thorough evaluation, a definitive diagnosis for RPL will be made in only 50% of patients. The following review of causes includes the evidence-based evaluation for RPL associated with each cause.

ANATOMIC CAUSES

Congenital and acquired uterine anomalies are found in 10% to 15% of women with RPL compared with 7% of all reproductive-aged women.[8,9] A uterine evaluation is widely considered an important part of the evaluation for patients with RPL and may include a hysterosalpingogram (HSG), saline infusion sonogram (SIS), 3-dimensional (3D) ultrasound, diagnostic hysteroscopy, or MRI.

Congenital uterine anomalies are associated with second-trimester losses and other obstetric complications, such as preterm labor, fetal malpresentation, and a higher rate of delivery by cesarean section. Although the role of uterine anomalies in

Table 1 Definitions of pregnancy and RPL	
Pregnancy	Clinical pregnancy documented by ultrasonography or histopathologic examination
Clinical miscarriage	Pregnancy loss before the twentieth week of gestation
Biochemical pregnancy	Beta Human Chorionic Gonadotropin hormone detected in urine or blood stream, but pregnancy loss occurs before it could be clinically documented
RPL: classic definition	Three pregnancy losses before the twentieth week of gestation and excludes ectopic, molar, and biochemical pregnancies
RPL: evaluation indicated according to ASRM	Clinical evaluation may proceed following 2 first-trimester pregnancy losses
Primary RPL	RPL in a patient who has never had a live birth
Secondary RPL	RPL in a patient who has had at least one live birth

first-trimester losses is debated, uterine cavity evaluation is widely considered a part of the evaluation for RPL.[10–15] Mullerian tract anomalies include unicornuate, didelphic, bicornuate, septate, or arcuate uteri. A review of several studies found that congenital uterine anomalies are present in 4.3% (range 2.75%–16.7%) of the general population of fertile women and in 12.6% (range 1.5%–37.6%) of patients with RPL defined as 2 or more losses.[16] A high rate of miscarriage occurred in patients with septate (n = 499, 44.3% loss), bicornuate (n = 627, 36.0% loss), and arcuate (n = 241, 25.7% loss) uteri. Surgical resection of uterine septums showed beneficial effects (n = 366, live birth rate 83.2%, range 77.4%–90.9%). All data came from retrospective reviews or observational studies.

The clinical management of patients with RPL with acquired uterine abnormalities, such as adhesions, polyps, retained products of conception, and fibroids, is debated. Submucosal fibroids may impede implantation because of the position, poor endometrial receptivity, or degeneration leading to increased cytokine production.[17] Intrauterine adhesions may lead to an increased risk of miscarriage because there is insufficient endometrium to support a developing pregnancy.[18] There is likely less biological plausibility to argue how endometrial polyps may impact implantation. There are no randomized controlled trials showing that surgical intervention decreases the subsequent miscarriage rate; however, the general consensus is that hysteroscopic correction of these defects should be considered[1] because of the potential impact on subsequent fertility, miscarriage, and pregnancy outcomes.

The options for uterine evaluation include HSG, hysteroscopy, SIS, and overall anatomy with 3D ultrasound or MRI. The selection depends on the availability and access for each provider and patient. The gold standard for uterine cavity evaluation is a diagnostic hysteroscopy; however, this is more invasive than an HSG or SIS. A SIS may be more accessible to some providers and patients, allows for the view of the ovaries and intramural uterine lesions, and avoids radiation. A uterine evaluation for RPL may stop with a normal cavity evaluation with HSG, SIS, or diagnostic hysteroscopy. However, if a congenital anomaly is suspected, additional imaging is needed. A congenital anomaly will be more fully characterized by 3D ultrasound or MRI because a full view of the uterus is needed to differentiate some anomalies (especially septate vs bicornuate). If a uterine anomaly is detected, one should consider evaluating the renal system because renal and uterine anomalies are often associated.[19]

ANTIPHOSPHOLIPID SYNDROME

The antiphospholipid syndrome (APS) is associated with RPL. Diagnostic criteria are outlined in **Box 1**.[20,21] Consensus statements agree that approximately 5% to 20% of patients with RPL will test positive for antiphospholipid antibodies (aPLs), although some report an incidence as high as 42%.[21,22] Laboratory assays have not been standardized,[20] which leads to high variability between laboratories and assays. The most widely accepted tests are lupus anticoagulant, anticardiolipin antibody, and anti-B2 glycoprotein I.[23] These antibodies have several detrimental effects on the developing trophoblast, including inhibition of villous cytotrophoblast differentiation and extravillous cytotrophoblast invasion into the decidua,[24–28] induction of syncytiotrophoblast apoptosis,[29] and initiation of maternal inflammatory pathways on the syncytiotrophoblast surface.[30–33]

The identification of aPLs and subsequent treatment of patients with RPL with these antibodies is highly debated. The aPLs are highly diverse among patients and results vary. With the exception of lupus anticoagulant, anticardiolipin, anti-B2-glycoprotein,

---

Box 1
International consensus classification criteria for APS

APS is present if one of the following clinical criteria and one of the laboratory criteria are met:

Clinical criteria

1. Vascular thrombosis

2. Pregnancy morbidity

   a. One or more unexplained deaths of morphologically normal fetuses after the 10th week of gestation by ultrasound or direct examination of the fetus

   b. One or more premature births of a morphologically normal neonate before the 34th week of gestation caused by eclampsia, severe preeclampsia, or recognized features of placental insufficiency

   c. Three or more unexplained consecutive spontaneous abortions before the 10th week of gestation with maternal anatomic or hormonal abnormalities and paternal and maternal chromosomal causes excluded

Laboratory criteria

1. Lupus anticoagulant present in plasma on 2 or more occasions at least 12 weeks apart or

2. Anticardiolipin antibody of IgG or IgM isotype in serum or plasma present in medium or high titer (>40 GPL (1 GPL unit is microgram of IgG antibody) or MPL (1 MPL unit is 1 microgram of 1gM antibody) or >99th percentile) on 2 or more occasions at least 12 weeks apart or

3. Anti-b2 glycoprotein-I antibody of IgG and/or IgM isotype in serum or plasma (in titer greater than the 99th percentile) present on 2 or more occasions at least 12 weeks apart

Abbreviations: IgG, immunoglobulin G; IgM, immunoglobulin M.

Data from American College of Obstetricians Gynecologists, Committee on Practice Bulletins-Obstetrics. ACOG practice bulletin No. 132: antiphospholipid syndrome. Obstet Gynecol 2012;120:1514–21; and Yetman DL, Kutteh SR. Antiphospholipid antibody panels and recurrent pregnancy loss: prevalence of anticardiolipin antibodies compared with other antiphospholipid antibodies. Fertil Steril 1996;55:540–6.

---

and antiphosphatidylserine, clinical assays for aPLs are not standard; routine screening is not warranted.[1] Testing for additional aPLs will increase the statistical probability of finding a positive test and possibly lead to unnecessary intervention.

The authors of the international consensus statement provide recommendations for several clinical events that should trigger testing for aPLs (see **Box 1**).[20] That group recommends testing patients with 3 or more unexplained spontaneous abortions before the 10th week of gestation. Unexplained spontaneous loss requires excluding maternal anatomic or hormonal abnormalities and paternal and maternal chromosomal causes. The group recommended screening for aPLs in the setting of a single unexplained loss of a morphologically normal fetus at or beyond 10 weeks' gestation.[20] In many cases, a miscarriage is diagnosed weeks after the pregnancy has stopped developing. A situation whereby a miscarriage is diagnosed after 10 weeks' gestation but ultrasound evidence is available that shows a pregnancy stopped developing earlier than 10 weeks would not warrant aPLs testing. An association between APS and preeclampsia has been suggested; in a combined analysis of 9 studies (n = 741), 17.9% of patients with severe preeclampsia had moderate to high levels of aPLs.[34–42] Thus, consider screening patients for aPLs who have a history of delivering a morphologically normal fetus before 34 weeks in the setting of severe preeclampsia or placental insufficiency (intrauterine growth restriction).[1]

The treatment of documented APS consists of low-dose aspirin (usually 81 mg daily) and heparin (usually 5000 units by subcutaneous injection twice a day) beginning with a positive pregnancy test.[43,44] The strongest evidence for treating APS is a live birth rate of 74.3% in patients treated (n = 70) with both aspirin and heparin compared with 42.9% (n = 70) with aspirin alone.[45,46] Low-molecular-weight heparin has not been established as an effective alternative.[47,48] Administration of prednisone does not improve outcomes and may be associated with an increased risk of gestational hypertension and gestational diabetes.[48] Multiple large randomized trials examining the use of heparin and/or aspirin in women with RPL not meeting strict criteria for APS have shown no difference in clinical outcomes.[43,44] Therefore, the use of heparin and aspirin should be limited to only women who have met both the clinical and laboratory criteria for APS.

THYROID FUNCTION

Thyroid dysfunction can be associated with poor obstetric outcomes.[49] Untreated overt maternal hypothyroidism (elevated thyroid-stimulating hormone [TSH] associated with decreased T4 levels) is associated with poor obstetric outcomes, including miscarriage, premature birth, low birth weight, and gestational hypertension.[50-55] Subclinical hypothyroidism (serum TSH elevated but normal serum free T4 levels) has been associated with preterm deliveries, increased neonatal intensive care unit admissions, and neonatal distress after delivery.[56] Some studies found that euthyroid patients with autoimmune thyroid disease (positive thyroid antibodies in the setting of normal TSH and T4 levels) have a higher risk of miscarriage and recurrent pregnancy loss.[57-59] Other retrospective studies failed to show a higher miscarriage rate in women with positive thyroid antibodies compared with those without these antibodies.[60] Inadequately treated maternal hyperthyroidism has been associated with preterm delivery, intrauterine growth restriction, preeclampsia, congestive heart failure, and fetal death but not specifically associated with RPL.[61]

Universal screening of healthy women for thyroid dysfunction before pregnancy is not currently recommended.[49] However, providers may screen patients who are considered high risk for thyroid dysfunction, including women with a history of miscarriage. Recommendations for targeted thyroid screening when planning pregnancy or in early pregnancy are summarized at the following link: http://dx.doi.org/10.1210/jc. 2011-2803.

Screening for patients with RPL may include TSH and thyroid peroxidase antibodies.[49] A randomized prospective study found higher pregnancy complications in women with TSH levels greater than 2.5 mIU/mL in the first trimester with and without the presence of thyroid antibodies.[62] Retrospective data support these findings,[63] and correction of hypothyroidism before pregnancy restores pregnancy outcomes to the rate seen in euthyroid women.[64,65] Some studies contradict these findings.[55,66]

Although the evidence varies, consensus by the Endocrine Society in the 2012 practice guidelines for the "Management of Thyroid Dysfunction during Pregnancy and Postpartum"[49] recommends the following:

1. Screen all at-risk women either before pregnancy or when newly pregnant when risk factors for thyroid dysfunction present (http://dx.doi.org/10.1210/jc.2011-2803).
2. Repeat the test to confirm the assay result if the prenatal TSH level is greater than 2.5 mIU/L.
3. Administer T4 replacement to achieve a prepregnancy TSH level less than 2.5 mIU/L.

4. If the TSH is 2.0 to 10.0 mIU/L, a starting dosage of T4 at 50 mcg daily or more is recommended.
5. T3 replacement is not recommended.
6. Monitor TSH levels approximately every 4 to 6 weeks with adjustments in doses or, at a minimum, once a trimester.
7. For patients who are taking levothyroxine before conception, increase replacement by 30% to meet the demands of the fetus by taking 2 extra doses per week.
8. Most women will return to their prepregnancy dose of T4 replacement after delivery.

The ASRM's guidelines for the treatment of RPL states that, although TSH values of 4.0 to 5.0 mIU/L were once considered normal, a consensus is emerging that TSH values greater than 2.5 mIU/L are outside the normal range and should be addressed in patients with RPL.[1]

OTHER HORMONAL CONDITIONS

Poorly controlled diabetes is associated with pregnancy loss.[67] High hemoglobin A1C levels (especially greater than 8%) have been associated with an increased risk of miscarriage and congenital malformations.[68–70] The increased risk in poorly controlled patients is likely associated with hyperglycemia, maternal vascular disease, and possibly immunologic factors. Well-controlled diabetes is not associated with an increased risk of miscarriage.[71]

Elevated levels of prolactin (hyperprolactinemia) have been associated with an increased risk of miscarriage.[1] Theories of this association involve prolactin's ability to alter the hypothalamic-pituitary-ovarian axis resulting in impaired folliculogenesis and oocyte maturation and/or its involvement in implantation in the luteal phase. Using a dopamine agonist (bromocriptine) to normalize prolactin levels before pregnancy in patients with a history of RPL (2 or more losses) improved pregnancy outcomes in one randomized trial (live birth rate 85.7% in the treated group compared with 52.4% in the untreated group).[72]

Progesterone in the luteal phase is essential for implantation and early pregnancy development. Defects in ovarian progesterone production are likely to impact the early success of a pregnancy. A shortened luteal phase has been associated with pregnancy loss in the past, but assessment and interpretation of an inadequate luteal phase is problematic.[73] The use of histologic and/or biochemical testing for diagnosis is unreliable and not reproducible.[74] Routine endometrial biopsy for luteal-phase dating is not recommended.[75] Some newer markers for endometrial receptivity are currently being investigated but cannot be considered part of a standard RPL evaluation until further evidence emerges.

Serum progesterone concentrations are not reflective of endometrial tissue levels of progesterone and are not predictive of pregnancy outcome.[76] Supplementing progesterone with exogenous progesterone does not decrease the risk of sporadic miscarriage.[77,78] However, in patients with 3 or more consecutive miscarriages, empirical progesterone administration may have some benefit.[72,79,80] The types of progesterone supplements vary; but in general, intramuscular injections and vaginal suppositories are the most widely used. Oral progesterone is ineffective at increasing uterine progesterone levels. Recommendations differ on the timing of empirical progesterone supplement. Traditionally, progesterone administration was given after ovulation in the luteal phase. Starting progesterone supplements after a positive pregnancy test may provide adequate pregnancy support and reduce costs, side effects, and the emotional toll of a delayed menses and negative pregnancy test.

INHERITED THROMBOPHILIAS

Thrombosis of spiral arteries within the placenta may affect perfusion and lead to late fetal loss, intrauterine growth restriction, placental abruption, or preeclampsia. Inherited thrombophilia disorders including factor V Leiden, prothrombin gene mutation, and deficiencies in protein C, protein S, and antithrombin may put a patient at an increased risk for late (second and third trimester) losses but have not been associated with recurrent first-trimester losses.[81,82]

Screening for inherited thrombophilias may be justified in patients with a personal history of thrombosis in a nonrisk setting (ie, not associated with surgery) or a first-degree relative with a known or suspected high risk of a thrombophilia.[1] Routine testing of women with RPL for inherited thrombophilia is not currently recommended.[21,83]

INFECTION

Some pathogens have been found more frequently in vaginal and cervical cultures of women with sporadic miscarriages. These pathogens include *Mycoplasma hominis*, chlamydia, *Listeria monocytogenes*, *Ureaplasma urealyticum*, Toxoplasma gondii, rubella, cytomegalovirus, herpes virus, and others.[84] No pathogens have been proven to cause RPL, and routine screening for infectious agents in patients with RPL is not recommended.[1,85] The use of empirical antibiotics in patients with asymptomatic RPL is not supported by randomized prospective studies.[1]

MALE FACTOR

The male contribution to miscarriage and RPL is highly debated. Some studies find a trend toward abnormal sperm morphology and RPL,[86–88] whereas other data do not support an association between any standard sperm parameters and RPL.[89] Sperm aneuploidy and DNA fragmentation have been studied in couples with RPL, but no strong association has been determined.[90] A single randomized controlled trial showed improved subsequent live birth rates after varicocelectomy in couples with RPL when the male partner has a significant varicocele.[91] A semen analysis and/or referral to a urologist may be informative in couples taking longer than expected to conceive, but no sperm testing should be considered a routine evaluation for a couple with RPL.[1]

ALLOIMMUNE FACTORS

Studies investigating the association of RPL with HLA typing, embryotoxic factors, HLA-G polymorphisms, antipaternal antibodies, decidual cytokine profiles, and natural killer cells have been inconsistent and nonreproducible.[1] Immunomodulation treatments designed to address these issues have not been proven to be effective.[1]

Treatments designed to develop immune tolerance, such as paternal white blood cell immunization (also known as lymphocyte immunization therapy), have not been shown to be effective at decreasing the risk of miscarriage.[92] Immunosuppressive treatment with intravenous immunoglobulin has also been proposed as a treatment of RPL but has been shown to be ineffective in randomized controlled trials.[93,94]

ENVIRONMENTAL AND PSYCHOLOGICAL FACTORS

Several environmental exposures are can be linked to the risk of sporadic miscarriage and, therefore, should be minimized in all couples considering pregnancy, particularly women with a history of miscarriage. Examples of these exposures are tobacco, caffeine, and alcohol. Although tobacco exposure has not specifically been linked to RPL, it is associated with adverse trophoblastic function, increased risk of sporadic miscarriage, and other poor obstetric outcomes.[95] Other exposures, including alcohol (3–5 drinks per week), cocaine, and caffeine (>3 cups of coffee per day), have been associated with an increased risk of miscarriage.[95–97] Obesity is linked to poor obstetric outcomes, including miscarriage[98] and RPL.[99] Obesity is an important risk factor to discuss because it is not only linked to the risk of euploid pregnancy loss but also to a higher recurrence risk in the setting of RPL compared with women of normal weight.[100]

RPL is extraordinarily impactful on a patient's emotional well-being, and awareness of the psychological needs of these patients is important. The grief and sense of loss for these couples can manifest itself in all aspects of personal and work life and may impact success with future pregnancies. Some small prospective studies have shown a positive influence in patients with RPL with the use of tender loving care (TLC) defined as psychological support with weekly medical and ultrasonographic examinations.[101,102]

GENETIC ABNORMALITIES IN RECURRENT PREGNANCY LOSS
Parental Balanced Translocations

Parental karyotype will identify chromosomal rearrangements that place couples at an increased risk of miscarriage. Parental balanced translocations affect 3% to 4% of couples with RPL. The most common types of balanced translocations are reciprocal translocations, which involve the exchanged of genetic material from one chromosome to another, and robertsonian translocations, whereby the long arms of 2 acrocentric chromosomes erroneously share a centrosome. Carriers of balanced translocations are typically asymptomatic, as they have the normal quantity of genetic material at all loci. However, during gametogenesis, the segregation of chromosomes may result in unbalanced gametes, which can lead to an increased miscarriage rate or ongoing conception with congenital anomalies. Although parental carriers of structural rearrangements have increased reproductive loss rates, similarly to patients with unexplained RPL, most carriers of parental translocation will succeed in having successful pregnancies without intervention.[103]

Preimplantation genetic chromosome screening (PCS) of embryos is one proposed therapy for carriers of parental translocations; however, well-designed prospective trials comparing expectant management with in vitro fertilization–preimplantation genetic diagnosis (IVF-PGD) or preimplantation genetic screening (PGS) have not been performed. Proponents have published several case series suggesting benefits, including fewer miscarriages, less emotional distress, and shorter time to successful pregnancy. However, these studies do not take into account the emotional and financial cost of a failed cycle or the time it takes to prepare for a PGS cycle in carriers of translocation. Fischer and colleagues[104] wrote one of the largest case series published to date on this subject. They reported on 192 couples with a history of 3 or more miscarriages undergoing IVF-PGD for either reciprocal or robertsonian translocations. Overall 35% of cycles had no suitable embryos for transfer, and the pregnancy rate per embryo biopsy cycle was 25%. The overall pregnancy loss rate in this cohort was 13%, and the live birth rate per cycle was 22%. Several smaller studies and reports either looked at individually or in summary do not show significantly different outcomes when day 3 biopsy and fluorescence in situ hybridization (FISH) is used.[104–107]

Scriven and colleagues[107] performed the only large intent-to-treat study in a population of carriers of translocations. They followed 59 couples with reciprocal translocations undergoing 1 to 3 cycles of PGS using cleavage stage embryo biopsy and FISH for their translocation. Only 110 of the 132 cycles started (83%) reached the biopsy stage, and 26% of cycles resulted in no eligible embryos for transfer. The overall live birth rate per initiated cycle was 20%. The investigators calculated that, based on their data, couples would have to undergo 3 cycles to achieve a 50% live birth rate. This study is particularly important because it calculates outcomes by intent to treat. This method showed that 40% of initiated cycles reach the embryo transfer. Their conclusion was that patients with a high risk of unbalanced viable offspring benefit from PGS, but that couples with lower-risk translocations may conceive more quickly without PCS and have a high rate of healthy offspring with spontaneous conception. They defined high risk of unbalanced offspring by personal or family history of an unbalanced live birth with congenital anomalies. Couples with balanced translocations benefit from genetic counseling to better understand their individual risk.

Very little data currently exist for the use of 24 chromosome screening of translocation carriers done after blastocyst biopsy. These data will be very helpful to couples with translocations. As we improve technology in this area, the live birth rate per transfer may increase. However, we must keep in mind that with extended culture and genetic screening there will be a higher rate of patients not reaching transfer. Patients willing to accept the risk and cost of PCS will likely see a significant reduction in miscarriage and reduction in the risk of unbalanced offspring. However, given the current literature, the chances of a healthy live birth per attempt are still low. Additionally, unbalanced live offspring are rare for most chromosomal rearrangements.

Aneuploidy and Miscarriage

Approximately half of couples with RPL will not have an identifiable cause for their losses.[12,13] The documented high incidence of chromosomal errors in first-trimester miscarriages has led to the theory that screening embryos before implantation for these errors may decrease the risk of a subsequent loss.

Most sporadic pregnancy losses in the first trimester result from random numeric chromosomal errors, specifically, trisomy, monosomy, and polyploidy.[6] Extensive research shows a consistently high rate of aneuploidy in analysis of pregnancy losses.[12,108–112] Approximately 60% of first-trimester pregnancy losses are associated with sporadic chromosomal anomalies.[6,113] Up to 90% of chromosomally abnormal pregnancies abort spontaneously,[6] but only 7% of chromosomally normal pregnancies abort spontaneously.[114] Miscarriage associated with chromosomal abnormalities increases with age.[115,116]

Analysis of pregnancy losses also shows a high rate of aneuploidy in some patients with RPL. The risk of aneuploidy increases with age such that up to 80% of miscarriages in patients with RPL who are older than 35 years.[116] The rate of aneuploidy in miscarriages increases with increasing maternal age. This association is seen in women with sporadic and recurrent miscarriages is not significantly different in women with RPL compared with women of similar in ages with sporadic miscarriage.[113] The type and frequency of chromosomal error is similar in patients with RPL to patients with advanced reproductive age.[117] The risk of aneuploidy in ongoing pregnancies may also increase with the number of previous miscarriages.[118]

Preimplantation Genetic Screening in Patients with Recurrent Pregnancy Loss

The evidence showing a high rate of aneuploidy found in sporadic miscarriages, and an increased rate of aneuploidy in patients with RPL, has provided a basis for suggesting embryo selection with PGS. PGS is a possible treatment option to decrease the risk of miscarriage in patients with unexplained RPL. The ability to provide genetic screening of embryos to patients with an increased risk of aneuploidy has been rapidly adopted in assisted reproductive technology, but the evidence remains limited.

Early investigations showed a higher rate of aneuploidy in the embryos from patients with RPL compared with controls using PGS for other reasons, such as X-linked disease.[119–121] One group using day 3 embryo biopsy and FISH for chromosome analysis showed a 70.7% aneuploidy rate in tested embryos from 71 couples with RPL (defined as 2 or more miscarriages) to a 45.1% aneuploidy rate in embryos from a control group of 28 couples doing PGS for sex-linked diseases ($P<.0001$). This group published a summary of their work in 2005 with 71 couples with RPL defined as 2 or more miscarriages compared with 28 couples undergoing PGD for sex-linked diseases.[122]

Munne and colleagues[123] compared the rate of miscarriage after IVF-PGS for patients with a history of 3 or more previous losses to their own expected loss rate based on age and number of previous miscarriages. A total of 58 patients with RPL (average age of 37.0 years) underwent IVF with day 3 embryo biopsy and FISH analysis for chromosomes 13, 15, 16, 17, 18, 21, 22, X, and Y. Patients with RPL experienced an average of 3.9 pregnancies before the intervention, of which 87% resulted in miscarriage. After IVF-PGS, 15.7% of pregnancies were lost ($P<.001$). The investigators also calculated the expected loss rate for each patient based on prediction parameters by Brigham and colleagues,[124] which uses a formula predicting the probability of successful pregnancy outcome based on the patient's age and pregnancy history. The expected miscarriage rate for 58 couples in the study was 36.5% based on Brigham's formula; however, the observed loss rate was 16.7% ($P = .028$). For patients 35 years old or older (37 patients), the expected loss rate was 44.5%; but the observed loss rate after IVF-PGS was 12% ($P = .007$). For patients with RPL who were less than 35 years old (21 patients), there were no differences between the expected and observed loss rate (29% vs 23%). The live birth rate per embryo biopsy was 40% for patients less than 35 years old and 34% for patients aged 35 years and older. This study suggested that women older than 35 years were more likely to benefit from PGS then younger women, which is consistent with studies that show patients with RPL who are younger than 35 years miscarry a higher percentage of euploid pregnancies than women older than 35 years.

Hodes-Wertz and colleagues[125] published a case series report on 287 IVF cycles from couples with unexplained RPL, defined as 2 or more losses, with PGS on cleavage stage biopsy (193 cycles), PCS on blastocyst biopsy (94 cycles), and chromosome analysis with array comparative genomic hybridization. The miscarrlage rate from these IVF-PGS cycles were compared with the expected miscarriage rate determined by (1) predictive parameters determined by Brigham and colleagues and (2) expected miscarriage rate in a control infertile population as reported in the United States to the Society of Assisted Reproduction Technology (SART). The overall aneuploidy rate for all 2282 embryos analyzed was 64.8%: 68.8% for cleavage stage embryos (1710 total) and 53% for blastocyst embryos (572 total). The average age of patients overall was 36.7 years $\pm$ 4.2 (36.5 $\pm$ 4.2 for cleavage stage biopsy and 36.9 $\pm$ 4.0 for blastocyst biopsy). The overall clinical pregnancy rate per embryo transfer was 55.2%, with a significantly higher pregnancy rate for blastocyst biopsy compared with cleavage stage biopsy (63.6% vs 50.4%, $P<.001$). There were 7 miscarriages overall (6.9%), which is less than the expected rate of miscarriage by Brigham and colleagues (33.5%) and SART (23.7%). There was a trend toward a higher miscarriage rate in cleavage stage biopsy compared with blastocyst biopsy (8.5% vs 4.7%), but this was not statistically significant.

The results of Hodes-Wertz and colleagues[125] look promising for the new technology; however, the data require careful interpretation. There were a total of 287 IVF cycles in couples with RPL, but the conclusions drawn are limited to certain groups. When reporting on pregnancy outcomes, only cycles with embryo transfers and pregnancy data are included (181 total); when reporting on miscarriage, only cycles with implantation are included (102 total). By excluding cycles that started but had no embryo transfer and cycles that were canceled before biopsy, intention to treat is lost, which overestimates the success rate of the PGS.

The technology has advanced rapidly in assisted reproductive technology and PGS. Early studies tested 1 to 2 cells from a day 3 or cleavage stage embryo and used FISH to test for euploidy; however, FISH allows for the diagnosis of only a few chromosomes. PGS is moving toward testing 4 to 5 cells from a blastocyst, which decreases the risk error because of mosaicism; 24 chromosome testing increases the detection of chromosomal abnormalities associated with miscarriage. The advances in technology seem promising. However, the costs, success rates, and number needed to treat with the use of PGS for individual patient groups have yet to be clarified.

Future research should be held to a high standard in order to provide the strongest evidence. First, miscarriage should be defined as a clinical loss by ultrasound evidence of histopathologic evidence because medical records could verify only 71% of reported miscarriages.[14] Second, although defining RPL as 2 or more losses may be beneficial clinically in order to identify treatable causes in women to prevent a third miscarriage, maintaining a distinction of 3 or more losses for inclusion criteria in research design would provide stronger evidence.[126] Third, intention-to-treat analysis must be used so that results are reported on all patients doing IVF with the intention of genetic screening of the embryos, not just the patients who have embryos suitable for transfer. Finally, the most challenging part of designing a compelling clinical study for patients with RPL will be finding an appropriate comparison group. The best evidence would be a randomized controlled trial of patients with RPL in which half of the patients had the intervention of IVF-PCS and the other half had no intervention beyond expectant management. With the possibility of a benefit of any intervention, finding a control group willing to forgo such treatment will be extremely difficult.

Furthermore, it must be stated that for any intervention in patients with RPL to be recommended, it must be shown to provide a higher chance of live birth beyond no intervention. IVF with PGS has medical risks and financial burdens to patients that must be justified before widespread use of this technology is offered as standard care. Given the current state of the literature, a provider must provide balanced and evidence-based counseling to patients with RPL. On one hand, IVF-PGS seems to decrease the miscarriage risk compared with natural conception; however, the live birth rate per started cycle is variable. Given this, the emotional and financial burden of IVF and PGS must be weighed against the estimated chances of live birth and the risk of subsequent miscarriage without this treatment. Patient preference for intervention, financial means, and social support will be important determinants of a patient's choice for or against treatment. The journey of RPL is challenging, and provider support throughout the process is essential regardless of a patient's choice for treatment.

REFERENCES

1. Practice Committee Opinion of the American Society of Reproductive Medicine. Evaluation and treatment of recurrent pregnancy loss: a committee opinion. Fertil Steril 2012;98:1103–11.

2. Ansari AH, Kirkpatrick B. Recurrent pregnancy loss. An update. J Reprod Med 1998;43:806–14.
3. Stirrat GM. Recurrent miscarriage. Lancet 1990;336:673–5.
4. Wilcox AJ, Weinberg CR, O'Connor JF, et al. Incidence of early loss of pregnancy. N Engl J Med 1988;319:189–94.
5. Edmonds DK, Lindsay KS, Miller JF, et al. Early embryonic mortality in women. Fertil Steril 1982;38:447–53.
6. Jacobs PS, Hassold T. Chromosomal abnormalities: origin and etiology in abortuses and live births. In: Vogel F, Sperlin K, editors. Human genetics. Berlin: Springer-Verlag; 1987. p. 233–44.
7. Knudsen UB, Hansen V, Juul S, et al. Prognosis of a new pregnancy following previous spontaneous abortions. Eur J Obstet Gynecol Reprod Biol 1991;39:31–6.
8. Harger JH, Archer DF, Marchese SG, et al. Etiology of recurrent pregnancy losses and outcome of subsequent pregnancies. Obstet Gynecol 1983;62: 574–81.
9. Acien P, Acien M, Sanchez-Ferrer M. Complex malformations of the female genital tract. New types and revision of classification. Hum Reprod 2004;19: 2377–84.
10. Stephenson MD, Kutteh W. Evaluation and management of recurrent early pregnancy loss. Clin Obstet Gynecol 2007;50:132–45.
11. Royal College of Obstetricians and Gynaecologists, Scientific Advisory Committee, Guideline No. 17. The investigation and treatment of couples with recurrent miscarriage. 2011. Available at: http://www.rcoag.org.uk/womens-health/clinical-guidance/investigation-and-treatment-couples-recurrent-miscarriage-green-top-. Accessed March 22, 2012.
12. Stephenson MD. Frequency of factors associated with habitual abortion in 197 couples. Fertil Steril 1996;66:24–9.
13. Jaslow CR, Carney JL, Kutteh WH. Diagnostic factors identified in 1020 women with two vs. three or more recurrent pregnancy losses. Fertil Steril 2010;93: 1234–43.
14. Christiansen OB, Nybo Andersen AM, Bosch E, et al. Evidence-based investigations and treatment of recurrent pregnancy loss. Fertil Steril 2005;83:821–39.
15. Rai R, Regan L. Recurrent miscarriage. Lancet 2006;368:601–11.
16. Grimbizis GF, Camus M, Tarlatzis BC, et al. Clinical implications of uterine malformations and hysteroscopic treatment results. Hum Reprod Update 2001;7:161–74.
17. Simpson JL. Causes of fetal wastage. Clin Obstet Gynecol 2007;50:10–30.
18. Pabuçcu R, Atay V, Orhon E, et al. Hysteroscopic treatment of intrauterine adhesions is safe and effective in the restoration of normal menstruation and fertility. Fertil Steril 1997;68:1141–3.
19. Hall-Craggs MA, Kirkham A, Creighton SM. Renal and urological abnormalities occurring with Mullerian anomalies. J Pediatr Urol 2013;9:27–32.
20. Miyakis S, Lockshin MD, Atsumi T, et al. International consensus statement on an update if the classification criteria for definite antiphospholipid syndrome (APS). J Thromb Haemost 2006;4:295–306.
21. Committee on Practice Bulletins—Obstetrics, American College of Obstetricians and Gynecologists. Practice bulletin No. 132: antiphospholipid syndrome. Obstet Gynecol 2012;120:1514–21.
22. Yetman DL, Kutteh SR. Antiphospholipid antibody panels and recurrent pregnancy loss: prevalence of anticardiolipin antibodies compared with other antiphospholipid antibodies. Fertil Steril 1996;55:540–6.

23. Opartrny L, David M, Kahn SR, et al. Association between antiphospholipid antibodies and recurrent fetal loss in women without autoimmune disease: a meta-analysis. J Rheumatol 2006;33:2214–21.
24. Adler RR, Ng AK, Rote NS. Monoclonal antiphosphatidylserine antibody inhibits intercellular fusion of the choriocarcinoma line, JAR. Biol Reprod 1995;53: 905–10.
25. Rote NS, Lyden TW, Vogt E, et al. Chapter 18: antiphospholipid antibodies and placental development. In: Hunst JS, editor. Immunobiology of reproduction. New York: Springer-Verlaf; 1994. p. 285–302.
26. Katsuragawa H, Kanzaki H, Iniue T, et al. Monoclonal antibody against phospha-tidylserine inhibits in vitro human trophoblastic hormone production and invasion. Biol Reprod 1997;56:50–8.
27. Di Simone N, Meroni PL, de Papa N, et al. Antiphospholipid antibodies affect trophoblast gonadotropin secretion and invasiveness by binding directly and through adhered beta2-glycoprotein I. Arthritis Rheum 2000;43:140–50.
28. Rote NS, Stetzer B. Autoimmune disease as a cause of reproductive failure. Clin Lab Med 2003;23:265–93.
29. DiSimone N, Catellani R, Caliandro D, et al. Monoclonal anti-annexin V antibody inhibits trophoblast gonadotropin secretion and induces syncytiotrophoblast apoptosis. Biol Reprod 2001;65:1766–70.
30. Vogt E, Ng AK, Rote NS. Antiphosphatidylserine antibody removes annexin V and facilitates the binding of prothrombin at the surface of a choriocarcinoma model of trophoblast differentiation. Am J Obstet Gynecol 1997;177:964–72.
31. Rand JH. The pathogenic role of annexin-V in the antiphospholipid syndrome. Curr Rheumatol Rep 2000;2:246–51.
32. Rand JH. The antiphospholipid syndrome. Annu Rev Med 2003;54:409–24.
33. Giardi G, Bulla R, Salmon JE, et al. The complement system in the pathophys-iology of pregnancy. Mol Immunol 2006;43:68–77.
34. Branch DW, Andres R, Difre KB, et al. The association of antiphospholipid antibodies with severe preeclampsia. Obstet Gynecol 1989;73:541–5.
35. Sletnes KE, Wisloff F, Moe N, et al. Antiphospholipid antibodies in preeclamptic women: relation to growth retardation and neonatal outcome. Acta Obstet Gynecol Scand 1992;71:112–7.
36. Yamamoto T, Yoshimura S, Geshi Y, et al. Measurement of antiphospholipid antibody of ELISA using purified bet 2-glycoprotein I in preeclampsia. Clin Exp Immunol 1993;94:196–200.
37. Dekker GA, de Vries JI, Doelitzsch PM, et al. Underlying disorders associ-ated with severe early onset preeclampsia. Am J Obstet Gynecol 1995; 173:1042–8.
38. Moodley J, Bhoota V, Duursma J, et al. The association of antiphospholipid antibodies with severe early onset pre-eclampsia. S Afr Med J 1995;85:105–7.
39. Allen JY, Tapia-Santiago C, Kutteh WH. Antiphospholipid antibodies in patients with preeclampsia. Am J Reprod Immunol 1996;36:81–5.
40. Yamamoto T, Takahashi T, Geshi T, et al. Anti-phospholipid antibodies in preeclampsia and their binding ability for placental villous lipid fractions. J Obstet Gynaecol Res 1996;22:275–83.
41. Van Pampus MG, Dekker GA, Wolf H, et al. High prevalence of hemostatic abnormalities in women with a history of server preeclampsia. Am J Obstet Gynecol 1999;180:1146–50.
42. Branch DW, Silver R, Pierangeli S, et al. Antiphospholipid antibodies other than lupus anticoagulant and anticardiolipin antibodies in women with recurrent

pregnancy loss, fertile controls, and antiphospholipid syndrome. Obstet Gynecol 1997;90:642–4.

43. de Jong PG, Kaandorp S, Di Nisio M, et al. Aspirin and/or heparin for women with unexplained recurrent miscarriage with or without inherited thrombophilia. Cochrane Database Syst Rev 2014;(7):CD004734.

44. Kaandorp SP, Goddijn M, van der Post JA, et al. Aspirin plus heparin or aspirin alone in women with recurrent miscarriage. N Engl J Med 2010;362:1586–96.

45. Empson M, Lassere M, Craig JC, et al. Recurrent pregnancy loss with antiphospholipid antibody: a systematic review of therapeutic trials. Obstet Gynecol 2002;99:135–44.

46. Empson M, Lassere M, Craig J, et al. Prevention of recurrent miscarriage for women with antiphospholipid antibody or lupus anticoagulant. Cochrane Database Syst Rev 2005;(2):CD002859.

47. Ziakis PD, Pavlou M, Voulgarelis M. Heparin treatment in antiphospholipid syndrome with recurrent pregnancy loss. A systematic review and meta-analysis. Obstet Gynecol 2010;115:1256–62.

48. Laskin CA, Bombardier C, Hannah ME, et al. Prednisone and aspirin in women with autoantibodies and unexplained recurrent fetal loss. N Engl J Med 1997; 337:148–53.

49. De Groot L, Abalovich M, Alexander EK, et al. Management of thyroid dysfunction during pregnancy and postpartum: an Endocrine Society clinical practice guideline. J Clin Endocrinol Metab 2012;97:2543–65.

50. Casey BM, Dashe JS, Wells CE, et al. Subclinical hypothyroidism and pregnancy outcomes. Obstet Gynecol 2005;105:239–45.

51. Glinoer D, Soto MF, Bourdoux P, et al. Pregnancy in patients with mild thyroid abnormalities: maternal and neonatal repercussions. J Clin Endocrinol Metab 1991;73:421–7.

52. Haddow JE, Palomaki GE, Allan WC, et al. Maternal thyroid deficiency during pregnancy and subsequent neuropsychological development of the child. N Engl J Med 1999;341:549–55.

53. Leung AS, Millar LK, Koonings PP, et al. Perinatal outcome in hypothyroid pregnancies. Obstet Gynecol 1993;81:349–53.

54. Man EB, Brown JF, Serunian SA. Maternal hypothyroxinemia: psychoneurological deficits of progeny. Ann Clin Lab Sci 1991;21:227–39.

55. Ablaovich M, Guiterrez S, Alcaraz G, et al. Overt and subclinical hypothyroidism complicating pregnancy. Thyroid 2002;12:63–8.

56. De Vivo A, Mancuso A, Giacobbe A, et al. Thyroid function in women found to have early pregnancy loss. Thyroid 2010;20:633–7.

57. De Carolis C, Greco E, Guarino MD, et al. Antithyroid antibodies and antiphospholipid syndrome: evidence of reduced fecundity and of poor pregnancy outcome in recurrent spontaneous aborters. Am J Reprod Immunol 2004;52: 263–6.

58. Stagnaro-Green A, Roman SH, Cobin RH, et al. Detection of at-risk pregnancy by means of highly sensitive assays for thyroid autoantibodies. JAMA 1990;264: 1422–5.

59. Iravani AT, Saeedi MM, Pakravesh J, et al. Thyroid autoimmunity and recurrent spontaneous abortion in Iran: a case-control study. Endocr Pract 2008;14: 458–64.

60. Negro R, Mangieri T, Coppola L, et al. Levothyroxine treatment in thyroid peroxidase antibody positive women undergoing assisted reproduction technologies: a prospective study. Hum Reprod 2005;20:1529–33.

61. Millar LK, Wing DA, Leung AS, et al. Low birth weight and preeclampsia in pregnancies complicated by hyperthyroidism. Obstet Gynecol 1994;84:946–9.
62. Negro R, Schwartz A, Gismondi R, et al. Increased pregnancy loss rate in thyroid antibody negative women with TSH levels between 2.5 and 5.0 in the first trimester of pregnancy. J Clin Endocrinol Metab 2010;95:E44–8.
63. Allan WC, Haddow JE, Palomaki GE, et al. Maternal thyroid deficiency and pregnancy complications: implications for population screening. J Med Screen 2000;7:127–30.
64. Vaidya B, Antony S, Bilous M, et al. Detection of thyroid dysfunction in early pregnancy: universal screening or targeted high-risk case finding? J Clin Endocrinol Metab 2007;92:203–7.
65. Tan TO, Cheng YW, Caughey AB. Are women who are treated for hypothyroidism at risk of pregnancy complications? Am J Obstet Gynecol 2006;194:e1–3.
66. Männistö T, Vääräsmäki M, Pouta A, et al. Thyroid dysfunction and autoantibodies during pregnancy as predictive factors of pregnancy complications and maternal morbidity in later life. J Clin Endocrinol Metab 2010;95:1084–94.
67. Jovanovic L, Knopp RH, Kim H, et al. Elevated pregnancy losses at high and low extremes of maternal glucose in early normal and diabetic pregnancy: evidence for a protective adaptation in diabetes. Diabetes Care 2005;28: 1113–7.
68. Greene MF, Hare JW, Cloherty JP, et al. First-trimester hemoglobin A1 and risk for major malformation and spontaneous abortion in diabetic pregnancy. Teratology 1989;39:225–31.
69. Miller E, Hare JW, Cloherty JP, et al. Elevated maternal hemoglobin A1c in early pregnancy and major congenital anomalies in infants of diabetic mothers. N Engl J Med 1981;304:1331–4.
70. Ylinen K, Aula P, Stenman UH, et al. Risk of minor and major fetal malformations in diabetics with high haemoglobin A1C values in early pregnancy. Br Med J (Clin Res Ed) 1984;289:345–6.
71. Mills JL, Simpson JL, Driscoll SG, et al. Incidence of spontaneous abortion among normal women and insulin-dependent diabetic women whose pregnancies were identified within 21 days of conception. N Engl J Med 1988;319: 1617–23.
72. Hirahara F, Andoh N, Sawai K, et al. Hyperprolactinemic recurrent miscarriage and results of randomized bromocriptine treatment trials. Fertil Steril 1998;70: 246–52.
73. Practice Committee of the American Society for Reproductive Medicine. The clinical relevance of luteal phase deficiency: a committee opinion. Fertil Steril 2012;98:1112–7.
74. Murray MJ, Meyer WR, Zaino RJ, et al. A critical analysis of the accuracy, reproducibility, and clinical utility of histologic endometrial dating in fertile women. Fertil Steril 2004;81:1333–43.
75. Coutifaris C, Myers ER, Guzick DS, et al. Histological dating of timed endometrial biopsy tissue is not related to fertility status. Fertil Steril 2004;82:1264–72.
76. Ogasawara M, Kajiura S, Katano K, et al. Are serum progesterone levels predictive of recurrent miscarriage in future pregnancies? Fertil Steril 1997;68:806–9.
77. Haas DM, Ramsey PS. Progestogen for preventing miscarriage. Cochrane Database Syst Rev 2008;(2):CD003511.
78. Goldstein P, Berrier J, Rosen S, et al. A meta-analysis of randomized controlled trials of progestational agents in pregnancy. Br J Obstet Gynaecol 1989;96: 265–74.

79. Oates-Whitehead RM, Haas DM, Carrier JA. Progestogen for preventing miscarriage. Cochrane Database Syst Rev 2003;(4):CD003511.
80. Daya S. Efficacy of progesterone support for pregnancy in women with recurrent miscarriage. A meta-analysis of controlled trials. Br J Obstet Gynaecol 1989;96: 275–80.
81. Dizon-Townson D, Miller C, Sibai B, et al. The relationship of the factor V Leiden mutation and pregnancy outcomes for mother and fetus. Obstet Gynecol 2005; 106:517–24.
82. Silver RM, Zhao Y, Spong CY, et al. Prothrombin gene G20210A mutation and obstetric complications. Obstet Gynecol 2010;115:14–20.
83. De Jong PG, Goddijin M, Middwldorp S. Testing for inherited thrombophilia in recurrent miscarriage. Semin Reprod Med 2011;29:540–5.
84. Penta M, Lukic A, Conte MP, et al. Infectious agents in tissues from spontaneous abortions in the first trimester of pregnancy. New Microbiol 2003;26:329–37.
85. American College of Obstetricians and Gynecologists. ACOG practice bulletin. Management of recurrent pregnancy loss. Number 24, February 2001. (Replaces technical bulletin number 212, September 1995). American College of Obstetricians and Gynecologists. Int J Gynaecol Obstet 2002;78:179–90.
86. Plouffe L Jr, White EW, Tho SP, et al. Etiologic factors of recurrent abortion and subsequent reproductive performance of couples: have we made any progress in the past 10 years? Am J Obstet Gynecol 1992;167:313–20 [discussion: 320–1].
87. Gopalkrishnan K, Padwal V, Meherji PK, et al. Poor quality of sperm as it affects repeated early pregnancy loss. Arch Androl 2000;45:111–7.
88. Carrell DT, Wilcox AL, Lowy L, et al. Elevated sperm chromosome aneuploidy and apoptosis in patients with unexplained recurrent pregnancy loss. Obstet Gynecol 2003;101:1229–35.
89. Hill JA, Abbott AF, Politch JA. Sperm morphology and recurrent abortions. Fertil Steril 1994;61:776–8.
90. Carrell DT, Liu L, Peterson CM, et al. Sperm DNA fragmentation is increased in couples with unexplained recurrent pregnancy loss. Arch Androl 2003;49: 49–55.
91. Mansour Ghanaie M, Asgari SA, Dadrass N, et al. Effects of varicocele repair on spontaneous first trimester miscarriage: a randomized clinical trial. Urol J 2012; 9:505–13.
92. Porter TF, LaCoursiere Y, Scott JR. Immunotherapy for recurrent miscarriage. Cochrane Database Syst Rev 2006;(2):CD000112.
93. Stephenson MD, Dreher K, Houlihan E, et al. Prevention of unexplained recurrent spontaneous abortion using intravenous immunoglobulin: a prospective, randomized, double-blinded, placebo-controlled trial. Am J Reprod Immunol 1998;39:82–8.
94. Hutton B, Sharma R, Fergusson D, et al. Use of intravenous immunoglobulin for treatment of recurrent miscarriage: a systematic review. BJOG 2007;114: 134–42.
95. Lindbohm ML, Sallmen M, Taskinen H. Effects of exposure to environmental tobacco smoke on reproductive health. Scand J Work Environ Health 2002; 28(Suppl 2):84–96.
96. Ness RB, Grisso JA, Hirshinger N, et al. Cocaine and tobacco use and the risk of spontaneous abortion. N Engl J Med 1999;340:333–9.
97. Kesmodel U, Wisborg K, Olsen SF, et al. Moderate alcohol intake in pregnancy and the risk of spontaneous abortion. Alcohol Alcohol 2002;37:87–92.

98. Boots S, Stephensen MD. Does obesity increase the risk of miscarriage in spontaneous conception: a systematic review. Semin Reprod Med 2011;29:507–13.
99. Metwally M, Saravelos SH, Ledger WL, et al. Body mass index and risk of miscarriage in women with recurrent miscarriage. Fertil Steril 2010;94:290–5.
100. Boots CE, Bernardi LA, Stephenson MD. Frequency of euploid miscarriage is increased in obese women with recurrent early pregnancy loss. Fertil Steril 2014;102:455–9.
101. Stray-Pedersen B, Stray-Pedersen S. Recurrent abortion: the role of psychotherapy. In: Beard RW, Ship F, editors. Early pregnancy loss: mechanisms and treatment. New York: Springer-Verlag; 1988. p. 433–40.
102. Stray-Pedersen B, Stray-Pedersen S. Etiologic factors and subsequent reproductive performance in 195 couples with a prior history of habitual abortion. Am J Obstet Gynecol 1984;148:140–6.
103. Stephenson MD, Sierra S. Reproductive outcomes in recurrent pregnancy loss associated with a parental carrier of a structural chromosome rearrangement. Hum Reprod 2006;21:1076–82.
104. Fischer J, Colls P, Escudero T, et al. Preimplantation genetic diagnosis (PGD) improves pregnancy outcome for translocation carriers with a history of recurrent losses. Fertil Steril 2010;94:283–9.
105. Lim CK, Jun JH, Min DM, et al. Efficacy and clinical outcome of preimplantation genetic diagnosis using FISH for couples of reciprocal and robertsonian translocations: the Korean experience. Prenat Diagn 2004;24:556–61.
106. Otani T, Roche M, Mizuike M, et al. Preimplantation genetic diagnosis significantly improves the pregnancy outcome of translocation carriers with a history of recurrent miscarriage and unsuccessful pregnancies. Reprod Biomed Online 2006;13:869–74.
107. Scriven PN, Flinter FA, Khalaf Y, et al. Benefits and drawbacks of preimplantation genetic diagnosis (PGD) for reciprocal translocations: lessons from a prospective cohort study. Eur J Hum Genet 2013;21:1035–41.
108. Daniely M, Avrium-Goldring A, Barkai G, et al. Detection of chromosomal aberration in fetuses arising from recurrent spontaneous abortion by comparative genomic hybridization. Hum Reprod 1998;13:805–9.
109. Ogasawara M, Aoki K, Okada S, et al. Embryonic karyotype of abortuses in relation to the number of previous miscarriages. Fertil Steril 2000;73:300–4.
110. Carp H, Toder V, Avirum A, et al. Karyotype of the abortus in recurrent miscarriage. Fertil Steril 2001;75:678–82.
111. Fritz B, Hallermann C, Olert J, et al. Cytogenetic analyses of culture failures by comparative genomic hybridisation (CGH)-Re-evaluation of chromosome aberration rates in early spontaneous abortions. Eur J Hum Genet 2001;9:539–47.
112. Sullivan AE, Silver RM, La Coursiere DY, et al. Recurrent fetal aneuploidy and recurrent miscarriage. Obstet Gynecol 2004;104:784–8.
113. Stephenson MD, Awartani KA, Robinson WP. Cytogenetic analysis of miscarriages from couples with recurrent miscarriage: a case-control study. Hum Reprod 2002;17:446–51.
114. McFadyen IR. Early fetal loss. In: Rodek C, editor. Fetal medicine. Oxford (United Kingdom): Blackwell Scientific; 1989. p. 26–43.
115. Hassold T, Chiu D. Maternal age specific rated of numerical chromosome abnormalities with special reference to trisomy. Hum Genet 1985;70:11–7.
116. Marquard K, Westphal L, Milki A, et al. Etiology of recurrent pregnancy loss in women over the age of 35. Fertil Steril 2010;94:1473–7.

117. Mantzouratou A, Mania A, Fragouli E, et al. Variable aneuploidy mechanism in embryos from couples with poor reproductive histories undergoing preimplantation genetic screening. Hum Reprod 2007;22:1844–53.
118. Kiss A, Rosa RF, Dibi RP. Chromosomal abnormalities in couples with history of recurrent abortion. Rev Bras Ginecol Obstet 2009;31:68–74.
119. Pellicer A, Rubio C, Vidal F, et al. In vitro fertilization plus preimplantation genetic diagnosis in patients with recurrent miscarriage: an analysis of chromosome abnormalities in human preimplantation embryos. Fertil Steril 1999;71:1033–9.
120. Simon C, Rubio C, Vidal F, et al. Increased chromosome abnormalities in human preimplantation embryos after in-vitro fertilization in patients with recurrent miscarriage. Reprod Fertil Dev 1998;10:87–92.
121. Vidal F, Gimenez C, Rubio C, et al. FISH preimplantation diagnosis of chromosome aneuploidy in recurrent pregnancy wastage. J Assist Reprod Genet 1998;15:310–3.
122. Rubio C, Simon C, Vidal F, et al. Chromosomal abnormalities and embryo development in recurrent miscarriage couples. Hum Reprod 2003;18:182–8.
123. Munne S, Chen S, Fischer J, et al. Preimplantation genetic diagnosis reduces pregnancy loss in women aged 35 years and older with a history of recurrent miscarriages. Fertil Steril 2005;84:331–5.
124. Brigham SA, Conlon C, Farquharson RG. A longitudinal study of pregnancy outcome following idiopathic recurrent miscarriage. Hum Reprod 1999;14(11):2868–71.
125. Hodes-Wertz B, Grio J, Ghadir S, et al. Idiopathic recurrent miscarriage is caused mostly by aneuploid embryos. Fertil Steril 2012;98:675–80.
126. Platteau P, Staessen C, Michiels A, et al. Preimplantation genetic diagnosis for aneuploidy screening in patients with unexplained recurrent miscarriages. Fertil Steril 2005;83:393–7 [quiz: 525–6].

Progesterone and the Luteal Phase

A Requisite to Reproduction

Tolga B. Mesen, MD*, Steven L. Young, MD, PhD

KEYWORDS

- Progesterone • Luteal phase • Luteal phase deficiency • Luteal phase support
- ART

KEY POINTS

- Luteal phase deficiency is a disease without a reliable diagnostic test, impairing clinical research and patient care.
- Exogenous progesterone is the primary agent for luteal support during assisted reproductive technology treatment; however, the best delivery method, protocol, and formulation are not yet known.
- Vaginal or intramuscular progesterone seem to be equivalent in terms of pregnancy outcomes after in vitro fertilization.
- The best route of progesterone supplementation after frozen embryo transfer is not yet established.

INTRODUCTION

The normal menstrual cycle can be divided into two phases: follicular and luteal, which are separated by ovulation and bookended by the first day of menstrual bleeding. The follicular phase is dominated by the development of the preovulatory follicle, resulting in estrogen-stimulated endometrial proliferation, whereas the corpus luteum (CL) of its namesake luteal phase produces progesterone, which inhibits endometrial proliferation and determines endometrial receptivity. Without both phases working in series, natural reproduction is not possible. This article focuses on the normal physiology of the luteal phase, investigates the controversy surrounding luteal phase defect, and describes the role of luteal phase support in assisted reproductive technology (ART).

The authors have nothing to disclose.
Department of Obstetrics and Gynecology, University of North Carolina at Chapel Hill, CB 7570, Chapel Hill, NC 27599, USA
* Corresponding author.
E-mail address: tolga_mesen@med.unc.edu

LUTEAL PHASE PHYSIOLOGY

In the natural menstrual cycle, the follicular phase culminates with the maturation of the dominant follicle. Increasing estradiol, secreted from the granulosa cells inside the dominant follicle, triggers a surge of luteinizing hormone (LH) from the anterior pituitary. The LH surge propagates a series of events, beyond the scope of this article, that result in the breakdown of the connections of granulosa cells comprising the cumulus oophorous, reentry of the oocyte into the diplotene stage of prophase I of meiosis, and eventual rupture of the follicle and extrusion of the oocyte into the pelvis. While the oocyte is captured by the fimbria and possibly fertilized in the fallopian tubes, the postovulatory, deflated, and eggless follicle can easily be forgotten. However, the remaining follicular cells play an essential role in facilitating reproduction and maintaining normal menstrual cyclicity by forming the CL.

Before ovulation, the granulosa cells of the dominant follicle begin their transformation into the CL by enlarging and becoming vacuolated.[1] The vacuoles take up the pigment lutein (from the Latin *luteus*, meaning "yellow") giving developing CL its characteristic yellow color. Before ovulation the granulosa cells are separated from the circulation by the basal lamina, necessitating nutrients and communications travel through gap junctions. With luteinization, the basal lamina regresses and the theca cells migrate into the forming CL. In addition, there is prompt neovascularization of the developing CL,[2] mainly under the control of vascular endothelial growth factor and fibroblast growth factor, which are upregulated in the luteinized granulosa cells.[3] The result of the impressive neovascularization is one of the highest blood flows per unit mass in the body,[1] a fact clinically apparent to a gynecologist managing a hemorrhagic CL.

Although the CL secretes many different hormones, the sex steroid, progesterone, is of primary importance because it is necessary and sufficient to transform the endometrium to a state receptive to blastocyst implantation and to maintain early pregnancy.[1] The production of progesterone by the luteal cells depends on the availability of its circulating cholesterol substrate and is facilitated by a low-level LH stimulation.[4] To accomplish steroidogenesis, the luteal cells develop into 2 morphologic appearances, small and large cells, with distinct functions.[5] The small cells, likely derived from the theca cells,[6] contain LH and human chorionic gonadotropin (HCG) receptors.[7] The LH receptor regulates low-density lipoprotein cholesterol receptor binding and internalization of the cholesterol.[1] The large luteal cells are thought to arise from the granulosa cells.[6] These cells have a greater steroidogenic capacity but lack the LH and HCG receptors needed to stimulate growth and provide cholesterol substrate.[8] The small and large cells are linked by gap junctions facilitating rapid transport of signals between cells, providing a mechanism by which the large luteal cells, devoid of LH receptors, respond to LH stimulation and provide the primary source of progesterone.

Multiple experimental designs and clinical experience in patients undergoing ART treatment illustrate the importance of tropic LH secretion to progesterone production from the CL. In one classic experiment, rhesus monkeys with an obliterated median basal hypothalamus, and, therefore, absent gonadotropin-releasing hormone (GnRH) secretion, were given exogenous GnRH pulses of a uniform amplitude and frequency via a mechanical pump. When the GnRH pump was active during the luteal phase, LH and progesterone were secreted. Within hours of discontinuing GnRH pulses, LH and progesterone levels were undetectable.[9] In women, lacking GnRH due to hypophysectomy, progesterone from the CL can be maintained with LH infusion.[10] In women undergoing in vitro fertilization (IVF) with pituitary downregulation (lacking significant LH production), early ovarian progesterone production can be stimulated with supplementation of HCG, an LH analog. Further, the profound and rapid variation in progesterone levels throughout the luteal phase closely mimics LH pulsatility in the human[11] and rhesus macaque.[12]

The individual CL seems to have a programmed lifespan independent of LH secretion. The normal lifespan of the CL is 11 to 17 days (mean 14.2 days) from the time of ovulation to the onset of menses.[13] If not rescued by HCG production from a newly implanted pregnancy, the CL will regress into an avascular scar known as a corpus albicans, via a process termed luteolysis.[14] Studies in rhesus monkeys have illustrated LH stimulation can be removed for up to 3 days without luteolysis. When it is reinstituted, progesterone production returns, which suggests luteolysis is not an LH-dependent process.[15] The process determining luteal phase length and degradation of the CL is still incompletely understood.

The CL can be rescued from luteolysis and continue progesterone production by rapidly rising HCG produced by the trophoblast of early pregnancy. Blastocysts grown in culture have been shown to produce HCG 7 to 8 days after fertilization.[16] Although an early pregnancy is essential to the survival of the CL, a functioning CL is also essential to early pregnancy survival. The latter is evident in a classic series of studies by Csapo and colleagues[17] who performed luteectomy in pregnant subjects. Luteectomy uniformly resulted in abortion if performed before 7 weeks gestation. If luteectomy was performed between 7 to 9 weeks, abortion was sometimes seen. Luteectomy after 9 weeks resulted uniformly in pregnancy survival. Additionally, pregnancy could be salvaged by progesterone supplementation after luteectomy. These findings dramatically illustrate the transition from the embryo's dependence on the CL to the placental trophoblast for support and emphasize the absolute requirement for progesterone.[18]

The studies described above, as well as many others, highlight the essential role of luteal progesterone in pregnancy establishment and maintenance. Given this essential role, it is undeniable that there must be a progesterone threshold below which pregnancy establishment and/or maintenance is impaired or prevented. Thus, it is critical for the clinician to understand and recognize an abnormal luteal phase and understand the available therapies in both ART and non-ART cycles.

LUTEAL PHASE DEFICIENCY

Luteal phase deficiency (LPD) is a condition of insufficient progesterone exposure to maintain a normal secretory endometrium and allow for normal embryo implantation and growth.[19] The condition was first described as a possible cause of infertility by Georgiana Seegar Jones[20] in 1949. This early, elegant study investigated the luteal phase of 206 ovulatory women with primary or secondary infertility. Some of these women were found to have a blunted rise in basal body temperature, decreased 48-hour urinary pregnanediol excretion, and/or endometrial biopsies with inadequate secretory changes, and labeled with LPD. Despite this early description and 65 further years of research, the understanding of LPD is still incomplete and controversy continues to surround its pathogenesis and diagnosis.[21]

LPD is sometimes clinically manifest by a shortened luteal phase lasting less than 9 days, from the day of ovulation to menstrual bleeding.[20,22,23] LPD is also suspected when spotting begins many days before mensuration without a structural or infectious cause. LPD has been implicated as a cause of irregular menstrual bleeding,[24] infertility,[25,26] and recurrent pregnancy loss.[23,27,28] However, despite the repeated association, a 2012 American Society for Reproductive Medicine (ASRM) committee opinion reminds readers that LPD has yet to be proven as a cause of infertility.[19]

The Dilemma of Diagnosing Luteal Phase Deficiency

Confusion surrounding LPD is the result of inconsistent and unreliable diagnostic criteria. In the initial description, Jones[20] provided clinical (shortened luteal phase), laboratory (decreased urinary pregnanediol), and histologic (endometrial biopsy) criteria for the diagnosis. Much of the research conducted since this initial description has used these methods singularly or in combination to identify affected individuals.

The normal luteal phase length from ovulation to menses ranges from 11 to 17 days with most luteal phases lasting 12 to 14 days. One proposed diagnostic criteria for LPD is a shortened luteal phase of less than 9 days.[29] However, a short luteal phase can occur in up to 5% of healthy fertile women with no significant increase in short luteal phase seen in the infertile population.[13,30]

Use of low luteal phase serum progesterone as a diagnostic tool for LPD is plagued by the pulsatile release of progesterone from the CL, echoing the pulsatile release of LH from the pituitary. Serum progesterone levels can fluctuate 8-fold in a 90-minute period during the midluteal phase and range from 2.3 to 40.1 pg/mL during a 24-hour period in the same healthy subject.[11] Because this rapid fluctuation traverses almost the entire range of luteal values, there can be no standard for appropriate luteal phase progesterone in fertile women[31] and, therefore, a single value can neither diagnose nor exclude LPD in patients. It is suggested that the sensitivity and specificity of the test can be improved by evaluating pooled samples from three separate blood draws in the midluteal phase.[31] However, the frequency and amplitude of progesterone pulses preclude sufficient precision. In the original description of LPD by Jones,[20] daily luteal progesterone was offered as the most accurate, yet clinically impractical, diagnostic test. Other investigators have suggested a 24-hour or 48-hour urinary pregnanediol glucuronide level to minimize progesterone fluctuations.[32] Remarkably, despite the clearly established barriers to its use, isolated serum progesterone concentrations are still used in the published literature to define biochemical LPD.[23]

The luteal phase biopsy, once considered the gold standard[33] for LPD diagnosis, has also been shown to be too imprecise to be clinically useful for most patients. The goal of this test, previously considered by many clinicians to be a standard component of the fertility evaluation, was to detect histologic changes in the endometrium that were out of phase with the cycle in regard to days after ovulation.[34] If the morphologic characteristics lagged more than 2 days behind the known luteal day, then LPD was presumed. In a study investigating histologic endometrial dating in healthy fertile volunteers, there was poor correlation between the actual cycle-day based on urinary detection of LH surge and histology report.[35] The study demonstrated a poorer precision in the timing of histologic features than had been described in previous studies using less rigorously timed biopsies. A large, multicenter, randomized trial designed to assess an association between and abnormal luteal phase biopsy and fertility failed to show usefulness. In this trial, 332 fertile women and 287 infertile women underwent endometrial biopsy in the midluteal to late luteal phase. Contrary to expectations, out-of-phase biopsies were more common in the fertile women compared with their infertile counterparts (42.2% vs 32.7%, $P<.05$).[36] Taken together, these studies provide strong evidence that histologic evaluation of the luteal phase biopsy to determine luteal phase adequacy is imprecise and cannot distinguish between infertile subjects and fertile controls.

The ASRM committee opinion sums up these issues succinctly, "There is no reproducible, physiologically relevant, and clinically practical standard to diagnose LPD or distinguish fertile from infertile women."[19] The poor performance of the diagnostic tools used significantly complicates the interpretation of 65 years of research based on these tools. It is important to point out, however, that a test that is too imprecise to determine a disorder in an individual, may allow enrichment of groups with and without a disorder when applied to a larger population. However, the uncertainty is clearly driving research toward molecular biomarkers that may be a more specific tool for the evaluation of inadequate progesterone action.[37]

Pathophysiologic theories of luteal phase deficiency

Two mechanisms have been proposed as causes of clinical LPD. The first and likely more common cause relates to the impaired function of the CL resulting in insufficient progesterone and estradiol secretion.[38] Impaired function can be the result of improper development of the dominant follicle destined to become the CL or aberrant stimulation of a normally developed follicle. Both mechanisms result in a CL with deficiencies in progesterone production. The second theory suggests an inability of the endometrium to mount a proper response to appropriate estradiol and progesterone exposure.[39]

Because the CL originates from the dominant follicles, it is logical to infer that abnormal development of the dominant follicle could result in an abnormal CL. Multiple studies have found a correlation between low follicular follicle-stimulating hormone (FSH) and LPD as defined by luteal phase progesterone secretion or luteal phase biopsy.[40,41] However, other investigators have reported a normal FSH profile in the setting of luteal phase defect.[42] Abnormal LH pulsatility has also been implicated as a potential cause of LPD. Experiments by Soules and colleagues[43] found some women with LPD have a fixed and increased LH pulse frequency throughout the early follicular phase compared with women with normal luteal function who have an accelerating LH pulse frequency approaching ovulation. It is suggested that an earlier increase in LH pulse frequency in the early follicular phase leads to decreased LH bioactivity in the luteal phase, decreasing progesterone secretion.[44] The importance of pulsatile LH and FSH is further evidenced by patients receiving GnRH agonists or antagonists during ART cycles. These medications can cause suppression of pituitary LH secretion for 2 to 3 weeks after discontinuation, resulting in decreased CL progesterone production and necessitating progesterone supplementation for optimal outcomes.[45]

Another potential form of LPD is an abnormal endometrial response to adequate levels of progesterone exposure. Usadi and colleagues[39] investigated normal, young research subjects who underwent modeled cycles, highly similar to endometrial preparation for donor oocyte recipience, except that progesterone levels were reduced to simulate LPD. These subjects underwent pituitary downregulation with a GnRH agonist and were supplemented with estradiol, to mimic the follicular phase, followed by estradiol and varying doses of progesterone to mimic the effects of the luteal phase on the endometrium. These investigators found that unequivocally low levels of progesterone produced a completely normal appearing endometrium on histologic evaluation. The findings suggest that lower levels of progesterone might not be the sole culprit in LPD and there may be other molecular mechanisms affecting abnormal responses to progesterone and, therefore, abnormal endometrial development and receptivity.

Treatment of luteal phase deficiency

Due to the incomplete understanding of the pathophysiology and lack of an accurate method to diagnose LPD, empiric treatment of suspected LPD cannot be completely evidence-based. Clinical studies of treatment regiments are faced with a catch-22: how to evaluate treatment in a disease that cannot be accurately diagnosed. Most studies have used improvements in surrogate markers, such as endometrial biopsy and progesterone level, to show treatment effect. Unfortunately all attempts to link these surrogate outcomes to fertility outcomes have been unsuccessful.[19] Although these limitations preclude effective study of treatment regiments, they do not designate treatment attempts as nonsensical. Instead, this is an area in which many treating physicians believe that the art of medicine plays a role and they continue to treat patients they suspect to be affected by a LPD. In this scenario, the risk of the treatment must be exceptionally small.

Before considering treatment of LPD, it is important to evaluate and treat underlying conditions, such as hypothyroidism and hyperprolactinemia, which can alter the hypothalamic-pituitary-ovary axis function, causing abnormalities in hormone production. If clinical suspicion over multiple cycles points to LPD as a cause of infertility or miscarriage, it is reasonable to consider empiric treatment to correct LPD. Two strategies, improving the follicular development and supplementing progesterone, have been used to correct suspected LPD and treat infertility or recurrent miscarriage.

Extrapolating from studies showing impaired luteal progesterone secretion with lower gonadotropins in the follicular phase, it is inferred that more robust or numerous mature follicles will improve luteal progesterone secretion from the CL, correcting LPD. Therefore, many clinicians treat suspected LPD by attempting to optimize follicular development and number using ovulation induction agents, including clomiphene citrate (CC), letrozole, or injectable gonadotropins. To the authors' knowledge, only one small study has investigated the effect of clomiphene in subjects with LPD (diagnosed by out-of-phase endometrial biopsy).[46] In this study, designed to determine if the number of mature follicles after 100 mg of CC on cycle days 5 to 9 had an effect on endometrial biopsy, 10 out of 18 subjects with previously out-of-phase biopsies had an in-phase biopsy after receiving 100 mg of CC. However, how many would have had the same without CC cannot be determined. In a small retrospective study of 23 women investigating the use of injectable gonadotropins in women with presumed LPD and recurrent pregnancy loss, a significantly lower miscarriage rate was seen in those using gonadotropins versus controls (15% vs 58%).[47] To date, there are no published studies evaluating the effectiveness of ovulation induction with letrozole in women with LPD.

Progesterone supplementation is suggested as a treatment of LPD. Although frequently used, there is no published evidence that it improves pregnancy outcomes in natural cycles.[19] Progesterone may be supplied as micronized progesterone or synthetic progestins. Given reports of teratogenicity associated with synthetic progestins[48] (that have since been disproven[49]), natural micronized progesterone has been the treatment of choice. Micronized progesterone can be potentially supplied orally, sublingually, rectally, as an oil-based vaginal suppository, an aqueous vaginal cream, or intramuscularly (see later discussion).

A retrospective study comparing the CC treatment to progesterone vaginal suppositories in patient with presumed LPD based on endometrial biopsy showed a 100% pregnancy rate in those treated with progesterone and an 81% pregnancy rate in those treated with CC after 1 year.[50] These groups were compared with a historical population control with a pregnancy rate of 93%, suggesting effectiveness of treatment of LPD. A meta-analysis evaluated 3 underpowered controlled trails that failed to show a positive effect of progesterone treatment of recurrent pregnancy loss in patients with LPD.[51] When the studies were pooled, the odds ratio (OR) for ongoing pregnancy after treatment with progesterone was 3.09 (95% CI 1.28–7.42), suggesting a beneficial effect of progesterone. Well-designed randomized trials are needed to definitively answer whether ovulation induction or luteal progesterone supplementation is beneficial for patients with LPD.

It is the authors' clinic practice to consider treatment in patients with a clinical suggestion of LPD, including infertility or recurrent miscarriage in women with a short luteal phase or intermenstrual spotting without an identifiable cause. We typically treat with ovulation induction agents (50 mg CC or 2.5 mg letrozole on cycle day 5–9) and/or 200 mg micronized progesterone in oil suppositories beginning 3 to 4 days after LH surge. In patients with recurrent loss, the progesterone supplementation is often given after the first positive pregnancy test. We do not treat suspected LPD with injectable gonadotropins, given the high cost and unacceptable risk of twins or higher order multiples. We acknowledge these treatments are not based on strong evidence; however, they are based on clinical interpretation of underlying physiology and come with few risks.

LUTEAL PHASE SUPPORT DURING ASSISTED REPRODUCTION

Treatments that encompass ART include IVF, intracytoplasmic sperm injection (ICSI), and frozen embryo transfer (FET). These treatments frequently result in either the transfer of an embryo into a woman who has undergone controlled ovarian hyperstimulation with subsequent oocyte retrieval or a woman receiving an embryo in a nonovulatory cycle (FET or fresh embryo transfer of embryos from donor eggs into a recipient). In both situations, there is an effective LPD. In the patients who are receiving embryos in nonovulatory cycles, the need for progesterone supplementation is easy to understand given the absent CL. These are cycles in which the natural cyclicity is absent or suppressed, and the endometrial effects of the follicular phase are mimicked with estradiol supplementation to cause a proliferative endometrium. To prepare the endometrium for implantation of the embryo, the luteal phase is mimicked by exposing the endometrium to progesterone. Timing the transfer of an embryo to the appropriate duration of progesterone exposure allows for successful implantation. It is also clear that the luteal phase following controlled ovarian hyperstimulation and oocyte aspiration is dysfunctional, a fact that has been recognized since the infancy of IVF.[52] However, the reason for this deficiency is still controversial.[53] Multiple explanations for this phenomenon have been reported and subsequently disputed. It was initially assumed that the LPD after IVF resulted from destruction of granulosa cells destined to become the CL during oocyte aspiration. This theory was questioned after no changes in progesterone levels or luteal phase length were seen after aspiration of the single mature follicle in a natural, unstimulated cycle.[54] The administration of HCG to mimic the LH surge in IVF has been implicated as a cause of LPD by inhibition endogenous LH secretion from the pituitary.[55] However, normal luteal phase length and pregnancy rates are routinely seen in women receiving HCG triggers in natural cycles or while undergoing superovulation and intrauterine insemination. Other investigators have posited that the LPD is the result of GnRH agonist used to downregulate pituitary LH secretion, suppressing LH secretion well into the luteal phase.[45] With the advent of GnRH antagonists, which clear quickly and do not cause long-term pituitary LH suppression, premature luteolysis and poor pregnancy rates were seen when used during IVF cycles without progesterone support,[56] illustrating prolonged GnRH agonist pituitary suppression cannot be the sole cause of LPD in women undergoing IVF. Currently, the most widely accepted theory of LPD after IVF states the supraphysiologic steroid hormones secreted by the multiple CL in the early luteal phase of an IVF cycle causes direct inhibition of LH secretion via negative feedback on the hypothalamic-pituitary axis.[56–58]

The optimization of ART success rates relies not only on the creation of high-quality embryos but also on the establishment of a receptive endometrium. During the past 35 years, since the first IVF pregnancy and subsequent first pregnancy from frozen embryos, significant research has been directed toward establishing the optimum supplementation of the luteal phase in both IVF and FET cycles, with a goal to maximize live births while minimizing patient discomfort and inconvenience.

Luteal Phase Support in In Vitro Fertilization

Multiple treatments options, including progesterone, HCG, and GnRH agonist, have been tested in luteal phase supplementation after IVF. A recent Cochrane systematic review has evaluated many of these options and will be referred to in the remainder of this article.[53] In a recent survey of ART providers by Vaisbuch and colleagues,[59] all of the 408 centers across 82 countries used some form of progesterone for luteal phase support, with none of the surveyed centers using solely HCG, a historical treatment option. This is a change from a similar survey conducted 3 years earlier in which 5% of the IVF clinics were using HCG as the sole agent for luteal support.[60] Although luteal HCG has a similar effectiveness to luteal progesterone in terms of pregnancy outcomes, the avoidance of luteal HCG is due to the increased risk of ovarian hyperstimulation syndrome with this medication.[53,61,62] Given the paucity of use, luteal support with HCG is not further considered in this article.

Progesterone supplementation is available in multiple preparations, including intramuscular, vaginal, oral, or in a newly developed subcutaneous preparation. In a 2014 survey of 284,600 IVF cycles in 82 separate centers, 77% of the cycles were performed with vaginal progesterone only and an additional 17% used vaginal progesterone in combination with oral or intramuscular progesterone. Just 5% used only intramuscular progesterone and 0.5% used only oral progesterone.[59] However, there were regional differences in the choice of progesterone preparation with 57% of North American cycles choosing intramuscular progesterone. Subcutaneous progesterone is still in the trial phase.

Oral micronized progesterone was the luteal support progesterone of choice in the 1980s; however, it has since proven to be a poor treatment option. Although the most convenient form of progesterone, micronized progesterone, has poor and inconsistent bioavailability. After ingestion, it is absorbed by the intestines, undergoes a first-pass metabolism by the liver, and is excreted by the kidneys, resulting in a bioavailability that is only 10% of intramuscular preparations.[63] Serum levels reach maximum in 2 to 4 hours and remain significantly elevated for only 6 to 7 hours,[64] requiring more frequent dosing. In a randomized, controlled trial, users of oral micronized progesterone had a significantly decreased implantation rate compared with users of intramuscular progesterone (18.1 vs 40.9%, $P = .004$).[65] In a second trial, when compared against vaginal micronized progesterone, the oral route once again resulted in a lower implantation rate (10.7 vs 30.7%, $P \leq .01$).[66]

Given the allure of an oral agent for luteal support, other oral agents have been studied to replace oral micronized progesterone. Dydrogestrone, is an oral progestin with improved bioavailability compared with oral micronized progesterone.[67] In one randomized, controlled trial, pregnancy rates were higher in women undergoing IVF using oral dydrogesterone for luteal support versus vaginal micronized progesterone (41.0 vs 29.4%, $P \leq .01$).[68] A second trial comparing the same agents showed similar pregnancy rates.[69] Another randomized, controlled trial compared oral dydrogesterone to micronized progesterone vaginal gel (Crinone 8%) and found similar pregnancy rates (28.7 vs 28.6%).[70] Another synthetic progesterone, chlormadinone acetate, was compared with intramuscular progesterone with no changes in pregnancy rates or implantation rates.[71] In the 2011 Cochrane review, analysis favored the use of synthetic progesterone compared with micronized progesterone for clinical pregnancy (OR, micronized progesterone use: 0.79, 95% CI 0.65–0.96).[53]

Intramuscular progesterone was first described as a form of luteal supplementation during IVF in 1985.[72] The use of intramuscular progesterone is associated with injection site pain, skin irritation, inflammatory reactions, and rare abscess formation.[73] Early randomized trials comparing intramuscular progesterone to vaginal progesterone showed superior pregnancy rates in the intramuscular group.[73,74] However, since this time, multiple other randomized trials using newer progesterone preparations have been conducted and a 2009 meta-analysis showed no difference between the 2 groups in pregnancy rates and ongoing pregnancy rates.[75] A 2011 Cochrane review showed no difference in pregnancy or live birth rate; however, it did find a difference favoring intramuscular progesterone in ongoing pregnancy rates.[53] Intramuscular and vaginal administration of luteal progesterone are now considered by most investigators as equivalent in terms of IVF pregnancy outcomes.

Vaginal preparations of progesterone have become the mainstay of luteal supplementation during IVF because of their relative ease of use and equivalence to intramuscular progesterone. Vaginal progesterone is typically available as a tablet, suppository, or 8% gel. Vaginal progesterone benefits from a first-pass uterine effect in which endometrial tissue concentrations are typically much greater than would be expected based on serum levels.[76] Pharmacy-compounded vaginal suppositories are typically discouraged in IVF cycles due to unreliable and variable progesterone levels.[77] In a large, multicenter, randomized, controlled trial, progesterone tablets (Endometrin 100 mg twice a day or 3 times a day) were compared with 8% progesterone gel (Crinone 8% gel) with similar pregnancy and live birth rates between the 3 groups (live birth rate, Endometrin twice a day 35%, Endometrin 3 times a day 38%, Crinone gel 38%, normal saline).[78] Vaginal progesterone is well tolerated by most patients although some dislike this medication because of higher cost than injectable forms, difficulty with administration, and/or vaginal discharge.

Recently, a water-soluble injectable progesterone complex (Prolutex) has been developed for subcutaneous administration.[79] A pharmacokinetic study of this compound demonstrated sufficient serum progesterone levels to allow clinical use in ART.[80] To date, 2 randomized noninferiority trials have been conducted. The first compared subcutaneous progesterone (Prolutex) to 8% progesterone gel (Crinone) as luteal phase supplementation during IVF with no difference in ongoing pregnancy rate (27.7 vs 30.5%, P = NS).[81] A second randomized trial compared subcutaneous progesterone (Prolutex) to vaginal progesterone tablets (Endometrin) with no change in ongoing pregnancy rate (40.8 vs 43.3%).[82] Common side effects related to the subcutaneous injection include injection site pain, bruising, inflammation, and edema.

There is currently no consensus on when to begin progesterone supplementation during an IVF cycle. The first dose of progesterone is typically administered between the between the day of retrieval to 2 days after retrieval with no obvious changes in pregnancy rates.[83,84] Insight into the timing of embryo transfer in relation to progesterone exposure can be gathered from an experiment by Prapas and colleagues.[85] Vaginal or intramuscular progesterone exposure before transfer of fresh embryos from donor oocytes was varied from 2 to 6 days and implantation and clinical pregnancy rates were highest in a narrow window of progesterone exposure (Fig. 1). Most surveyed clinics (80.1%) begin progesterone supplementation on the day of egg retrieval.[59] In addition there is no consensus on the duration of progesterone use. A recent meta-analysis of 6 eligible studies and 1201 randomized subjects concluded there may be no additional benefit of progesterone supplementation

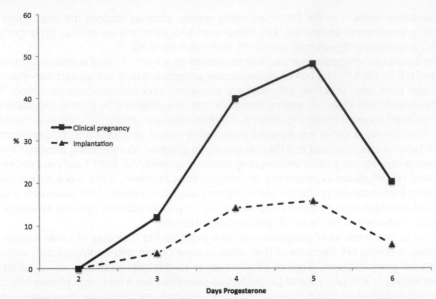

Fig. 1. Effect of days of progesterone exposure on implantation and pregnancy rates after cleavage-stage embryo transfer from donor oocytes. (*Data from* Prapas Y, Prapas N, Jones EE, et al. The window for embryo transfer in oocyte donation cycles depends on the duration of progesterone therapy. Hum Reprod 1998;13(3):720–3.)

beyond the first positive HCG value, showing no difference in live birth (risk ratio [RR]: 0.95, CI 0.86–1.05), ongoing pregnancy (RR: 0.97, CI 0.90–1.05), or miscarriage (RR: 1.01, CI 0.74–1.38).[86] Despite these data, most surveyed clinics (72%) continue progesterone until 8 weeks or more of pregnancy and only 15% discontinue progesterone after detection of beta HCG.[59]

Adjuvants to progesterone supplementation to increase IVF pregnancy rates have been widely discussed in the literature. The CL is not only a source of progesterone but also produces estradiol, along with many nonsteroidal hormones. Therefore, it has been suggested luteal support should include estradiol supplementation.[87] A 2008 meta-analysis identified 4 randomized studies evaluating estradiol supplementation in the luteal phase and found no difference between clinical pregnancy (587 subjects, RR: 0.94, CI 0.78–1.13) and live birth (527 subjects, RR: 0.96, CI 0.77–1.21).[88] In the 2011 Cochrane review, progesterone plus estradiol did not perform any better than progesterone in terms of biochemical pregnancy, clinical pregnancy, or live birth. However, when a subgroup analysis of clinical pregnancy was performed, progesterone alone performed worse then progesterone plus transdermal estradiol (OR: 0.50, CI 0.31–0.82), suggesting route of estradiol administration may play a role.[53]

Another suggested adjuvant to progesterone supplementation is a single dose of GnRH agonist 5 to 6 days after oocyte retrieval. It is hypothesized the GnRH agonist may support the CL by stimulating LH secretion for the pituitary but also may have effects on the endometrial GnRH receptors or direct effects on the embryo.[89] A 2010 meta-analysis[90] evaluated 5 randomized, controlled trials investigating luteal phase GnRH agonist[91–95] in both long and GnRH-antagonist protocols. When data were pooled, there was an increased pregnancy rate in cycles in which a single dose of luteal GnRH agonist was given 5 to 6 days after oocyte retrieval (42.4 vs 35.7%, OR: 1.33, 95% CI 1.08–1.64). A subgroup analysis was performed and pregnancy rate was significantly higher with luteal GnRH agonist used in a GnRH antagonist stimulation compared with the long protocol. Similarly, the recent Cochrane review showed increased pregnancy, ongoing-pregnancy, and live birth rates in subjects receiving luteal GnRH agonists.[53] Despite promising early evidence, additional study is needed given the lack of clear biologic mechanism before wide acceptance of this practice.

Luteal Phase Progesterone During Frozen Embryo Transfer and Donor or Recipient Cycles

Data from IVF cycles should not be extrapolated to FET or donor or recipient cycles because, unlike IVF cycles, there is no formed CL, thus no endogenous source of progesterone. In these cycles, exogenous estradiol is typically used to proliferate the endometrium, then exogenous progesterone is added to induce secretory changes in preparation for implantation. Intramuscular progesterone is typically used for this purpose in the United States, whereas in Europe vaginal progesterone is preferred.[96] Unfortunately, there are a paucity of data on this topic and, therefore, treatment decisions are based on limited information. Two small, prospective, randomized trials from the same group showed no difference in ongoing pregnancy rate when comparing intramuscular progesterone to vaginal progesterone in recipients of donor oocytes.[97,98] In addition, a retrospective study of donor oocyte recipients[99] and another retrospective study of subjects receiving donor and autologous frozen blastocysts[100] showed no difference in implantation, clinical pregnancy, or live birth rates. However, 2 other retrospective studies of women undergoing FET illustrated a deceased live birth rate in subjects receiving vaginal progesterone (24.4 vs 39.1%)[101] and (22.8 vs 34.5%).[102] The timing of progesterone exposure in FET and donor cycles has not been fully studied; however, a review of luteal progesterone during FET cycles was performed by Nawroth and Ludwig[103] and concluded cleavage-stage embryos should not be transferred before 3 to 4 days of progesterone treatment. In the clinical studies mentioned above,[97-102] cleavage-stage embryos were transferred on the fourth day of progesterone exposure and blastocyst were transferred on the sixth day of progesterone exposure.

SUMMARY

Progesterone production from the CL is critical for natural reproduction and progesterone supplementation seems to be an important aspect of any ART treatment. LPD in natural cycles is a plausible cause of infertility and pregnancy loss, although there is no adequate diagnostic test. Future research should concentrate on establishing thresholds of progesterone dose and timing for fertile and infertile women, as well as on a precise and accurate diagnostic test.

REFERENCES

1. Fritz MA, Speroff L. Clinical gynecologic endocrinology and infertility. Philadelphia: Lippincott Williams & Wilkins; 2012.
2. McClure N, Macpherson AM, Healy DL, et al. An immunohistochemical study of the vascularization of the human Graafian follicle. Hum Reprod 1994;9(8): 1401–5.
3. Anasti JN, Kalantaridou SN, Kimzey LM, et al. Human follicle fluid vascular endothelial growth factor concentrations are correlated with luteinization in spontaneously developing follicles. Hum Reprod 1998;13(5):1144–7.

4. Barbieri RL. The endocrinology of the menstrual cycle. Methods Mol Biol 2014; 1154:145–69 (Chapter 7).
5. Ohara A, Mori T, Taii S, et al. Functional differentiation in steroidogenesis of two types of luteal cells isolated from mature human corpora lutea of menstrual cycle. J Clin Endocrinol Metab 1987;65(6):1192–200.
6. Fujiwara H, Ueda M, Hattori N, et al. A differentiation antigen of human large luteal cells in corpora lutea of the menstrual cycle and early pregnancy. Biol Reprod 1996;54(6):1173–83.
7. Brannian JD, Stouffer RL. Progesterone production by monkey luteal cell subpopulations at different stages of the menstrual cycle: changes in agonist responsiveness. Biol Reprod 1991;44(1):141–9.
8. Retamales I, Carrasco I, Troncoso JL, et al. Morpho-functional study of human luteal cell subpopulations. Hum Reprod 1994;9(4):591–6.
9. Hutchison JS, Zeleznik AJ. The rhesus monkey corpus luteum is dependent on pituitary gonadotropin secretion throughout the luteal phase of the menstrual cycle. Endocrinology 1984;115(5):1780–6.
10. Vande Wiele RL, Bogumil J, Dyrenfurth I, et al. Mechanisms regulating the menstrual cycle in women. Recent Prog Horm Res 1970;26:63–103.
11. Filicori M, Butler JP, Crowley WF. Neuroendocrine regulation of the corpus luteum in the human. Evidence for pulsatile progesterone secretion. J Clin Invest 1984;73(6):1638–47.
12. Ellinwood WE. Changing frequency of pulsatile luteinizing hormone and progesterone secretion during the luteal phase of the menstrual cycle of rhesus monkeys. Biol Reprod 1984;31(4):714–22.
13. Lenton EA, Landgren BM, Sexton L. Normal variation in the length of the luteal phase of the menstrual cycle: identification of the short luteal phase. Br J Obstet Gynaecol 1984;91(7):685–9.
14. Strauss JF III, Barbieri RL. Yen & Jaffe's reproductive endocrinology: physiology, pathophysiology, and clinical management. Philadelphia: Elsevier; 2013.
15. Filicori M, Santoro N, Merriam GR, et al. Characterization of the physiological pattern of episodic gonadotropin secretion throughout the human menstrual cycle. J Clin Endocrinol Metab 1986;62(6):1136–44.
16. Lopata A, Hay DL. The surplus human embryo: its potential for growth, blastulation, hatching, and human chorionic gonadotropin production in culture. Fertil Steril 1989;51(6):984–91.
17. Csapo AI, Pulkkinen MO, Ruttner B, et al. The significance of the human corpus luteum in pregnancy maintenance. Am J Obstet Gynecol 1972;112(8):1061–7.
18. Csapo AI, Pulkkinen MO, Wiest WG. Effects of luteectomy and progesterone replacement therapy in early pregnant patients. Am J Obstet Gynecol 1973; 115(6):759–65.
19. Practice Committee of the American Society for Reproductive Medicine. The clinical relevance of luteal phase deficiency: a committee opinion. Fertil Steril 2012;98(5):1112–7.
20. Jones GS. Some newer aspects of the management of infertility. JAMA 1949; 141(16):1123–9.
21. Jones GS. Luteal phase defect. Curr Opin Obstet Gynecol 1991;3(5):641–8.
22. Sonntag B, Ludwig M. An integrated view on the luteal phase: diagnosis and treatment in subfertility. Clin Endocrinol (Oxf) 2012;77(4):500–7.
23. Schliep KC, Mumford SL, Hammoud AO, et al. Luteal phase deficiency in regularly menstruating women: prevalence and overlap in identification based on clinical and biochemical diagnostic criteria. J Clin Endocrinol Metab 2014;99(6):E1007–14.

24. Muechler EK, Huang KE, Zongrone J. Superovulation of habitual aborters with subtle luteal phase deficiency. Int J Fertil 1987;32(5):359–65.
25. Moszkowski E, Woodruff JD, Jones GE. The inadequate luteal phase. Am J Obstet Gynecol 1962;83:363–72.
26. Blacker CM, Ginsburg KA, Leach RE, et al. Unexplained infertility: evaluation of the luteal phase; results of the National Center for Infertility Research at Michigan. Fertil Steril 1997;67(3):437–42.
27. Swyer GI, Daley D. Progesterone implantation in habitual abortion. Br Med J 1953;1(4819):1073–7.
28. Smith ML, Schust DJ. Endocrinology and recurrent early pregnancy loss. Semin Reprod Med 2011;29(6):482–90.
29. Smith SK, Lenton EA, Landgren BM, et al. The short luteal phase and infertility. Br J Obstet Gynaecol 1984;91(11):1120–2.
30. Strott CA, Cargille CM, Ross GT, et al. The short luteal phase. Obstet Gynecol Surv 1970;25(8):775–7.
31. Jordan J, Craig K, Clifton DK, et al. Luteal phase defect: the sensitivity and specificity of diagnostic methods in common clinical use. Fertil Steril 1994; 62(1):54–62.
32. Santoro N, Goldsmith LT, Heller D, et al. Luteal progesterone relates to histological endometrial maturation in fertile women. J Clin Endocrinol Metab 2000; 85(11):4207–11.
33. Noyes RW, Hertig AT, Rock J. Dating the endometrial biopsy. Am J Obstet Gynecol 1975;122(2):262–3.
34. Wentz AC. Endometrial biopsy in the evaluation of infertility. Fertil Steril 1980; 33(2):121–4.
35. Murray MJ, Meyer WR, Zaino RJ, et al. A critical analysis of the accuracy, reproducibility, and clinical utility of histologic endometrial dating in fertile women. Fertil Steril 2004;81(5):1333–43.
36. Coutifaris C, Myers ER, Guzick DS, et al. Histological dating of timed endometrial biopsy tissue is not related to fertility status. Fertil Steril 2004;82(5):1264–72.
37. Young SL, Lessey BA. Progesterone function in human endometrium: clinical perspectives. Semin Reprod Med 2010;28:5–16.
38. Boutzios G, Karalaki M, Zapanti E. Common pathophysiological mechanisms involved in luteal phase deficiency and polycystic ovary syndrome. Impact on fertility. Endocrine 2013;43(2):314–7.
39. Usadi RS, Groll JM, Lessey BA, et al. Endometrial development and function in experimentally induced luteal phase deficiency. J Clin Endocrinol Metab 2008; 93(10):4058–64.
40. Aksel S. Sporadic and recurrent luteal phase defects in cyclic women: comparison with normal cycles. Fertil Steril 1980;33(4):372–7.
41. Cook CL, Rao CV, Yussman MA. Plasma gonadotropin and sex steroid hormone levels during early, midfollicular, and midluteal phases of women with luteal phase defects. Fertil Steril 1983;40(1):45–8.
42. Grunfeld L, Sandler B, Fox J, et al. Luteal phase deficiency after completely normal follicular and periovulatory phases. Fertil Steril 1989;52(6):919–23.
43. Soules MR, Clifton DK, Cohen NL, et al. Luteal phase deficiency: abnormal gonadotropin and progesterone secretion patterns. J Clin Endocrinol Metab 1989;69(4):813–20.
44. Miller PB, Soules MR. Luteal phase deficiency: pathophysiology, diagnosis, and treatment. In: Gynecology and obstetrics, vol. 5. Global Libr Women's Med. London: David G.T. Bloomer; 2009.

45. Smitz J, Erard P, Camus M, et al. Pituitary gonadotrophin secretory capacity during the luteal phase in superovulation using GnRH-agonists and HMG in a desensitization or flare-up protocol. Hum Reprod 1992;7(9):1225–9.
46. Guzick DS, Zeleznik A. Efficacy of clomiphene citrate in the treatment of luteal phase deficiency: quantity versus quality of preovulatory follicles. Fertil Steril 1990;54(2):206–10.
47. Li TC, Dinga SH, Anstie B, et al. Use of human menopausal gonadotropins in the treatment of endometrial defects associated with recurrent miscarriage: preliminary report. Fertil Steril 2001;75(2):434–7.
48. Burstein R, Wasserman HC. The effect of Provera on the fetus. Obstet Gynecol 1964;23(6):931.
49. Katz Z, Lancet M, Skornik J, et al. Teratogenicity of progestogens given during the first trimester of pregnancy. Obstet Gynecol Surv 1985;40(11):697–8.
50. Murray DL, Reich L, Adashi EY. Oral clomiphene citrate and vaginal progesterone suppositories in the treatment of luteal phase dysfunction: a comparative study. Fertil Steril 1989;51(1):35–41.
51. Daya S. Efficacy of progesterone support for pregnancy in women with recurrent miscarriage. A meta-analysis of controlled trials. Br J Obstet Gynaecol 1989; 96(3):275–80.
52. Edwards RG, Steptoe PC, Purdy JM. Establishing full-term human pregnancies using cleaving embryos grown in vitro. Br J Obstet Gynaecol 1980;87(9):737–56.
53. van der Linden M, Buckingham K, Farquhar C, et al. Luteal phase support for assisted reproduction cycles. Cochrane Database Syst Rev 2011;(10):CD009154.
54. Kerin JF, Broom TJ, Ralph MM, et al. Human luteal phase function following oocyte aspiration from the immediately preovular graafian follicle of spontaneous ovular cycles. Br J Obstet Gynaecol 1981;88(10):1021–8.
55. Miyake A, Aono T, Kinugasa T, et al. Suppression of serum levels of luteinizing hormone by short- and long-loop negative feedback in ovariectomized women. J Endocrinol 1979;80(3):353–6.
56. Beckers NG, Macklon NS, Eijkemans MJ, et al. Nonsupplemented luteal phase characteristics after the administration of recombinant human chorionic gonadotropin, recombinant luteinizing hormone, or gonadotropin-releasing hormone (GnRH) agonist to induce final oocyte maturation in in vitro fertilization patients after ovarian stimulation with recombinant follicle-stimulating hormone and GnRH antagonist cotreatment. J Clin Endocrinol Metab 2003;88(9):4186–92.
57. Fauser BC, Devroey P. Reproductive biology and IVF: ovarian stimulation and luteal phase consequences. Trends Endocrinol Metab 2003;14(5):236–42.
58. Fatemi HM. The luteal phase after 3 decades of IVF: what do we know? Reprod Biomed Online 2009;19:1–13.
59. Vaisbuch E, de Ziegler D, Leong M, et al. Luteal-phase support in assisted reproduction treatment: real-life practices reported worldwide by an updated website-based survey. Reprod Biomed Online 2014;28(3):330–5.
60. Vaisbuch E, Leong M, Shoham Z. Progesterone support in IVF: is evidence-based medicine translated to clinical practice? A worldwide web-based survey. Reprod Biomed Online 2012;25(2):139–45.
61. Daya S, Gunby J. Luteal phase support in assisted reproduction cycles. Cochrane Database Syst Rev 2004;3:CD004830.
62. Practice Committee of American Society for Reproductive Medicine in collaboration with Society for Reproductive Endocrinology and Infertility. Progesterone supplementation during the luteal phase and in early pregnancy in the treatment of infertility: an educational bulletin. Fertil Steril 2008;90(5):S150–3.

63. Simon JA, Robinson DE, Andrews MC, et al. The absorption of oral micronized progesterone: the effect of food, dose proportionality, and comparison with intramuscular progesterone. Fertil Steril 1993;60(1):26–33.

64. Maxson WS, Hargrove JT. Bioavailability of oral micronized progesterone. Fertil Steril 1985;44(5):622–6.

65. Licciardi FL, Kwiatkowski A, Noyes NL, et al. Oral versus intramuscular progesterone for in vitro fertilization: a prospective randomized study. Fertil Steril 1999; 71(4):614–8.

66. Friedler S, Raziel A, Schachter M, et al. Luteal support with micronized progesterone following in-vitro fertilization using a down-regulation protocol with gonadotrophin-releasing hormone agonist: a comparative study between vaginal and oral administration. Hum Reprod 1999;14(8):1944–8.

67. Coelingh Bennink HJ, Boerrigter PJ. Use of dydrogesterone as a progestogen for oral contraception. Steroids 2003;68(10–13):927–9.

68. Patki A, Pawar VC. Modulating fertility outcome in assisted reproductive technologies by the use of dydrogesterone. Gynecol Endocrinol 2007;23(Suppl 1): 68–72.

69. Chakravarty BN, Shirazee HH, Dam P, et al. Oral dydrogesterone versus intra-vaginal micronised progesterone as luteal phase support in assisted reproductive technology (ART) cycles: results of a randomised study. J Steroid Biochem Mol Biol 2005;97(5):416–20.

70. Ganesh A, Chakravorty N, Mukherjee R, et al. Comparison of oral dydrogestrone with progesterone gel and micronized progesterone for luteal support in 1,373 women undergoing in vitro fertilization: a randomized clinical study. Fertil Steril 2011;95(6):1961–5.

71. Iwase A, Ando H, Toda S, et al. Oral progestogen versus intramuscular progesterone for luteal support after assisted reproductive technology treatment: a prospective randomized study. Arch Gynecol Obstet 2008;277(4):319–24.

72. Leeton J, Trounson A, Jessup D. Support of the luteal phase in in vitro fertilization programs: results of a controlled trial with intramuscular Proluton. J In Vitro Fert Embryo Transf 1985;2(3):166–9.

73. Propst AM, Hill JA, Ginsburg ES, et al. A randomized study comparing Crinone 8% and intramuscular progesterone supplementation in in vitro fertilization-embryo transfer cycles. Fertil Steril 2001;76(6):1144–9.

74. Perino M, Brigandi FG, Abate FG, et al. Intramuscular versus vaginal progesterone in assisted reproduction: a comparative study. Clin Exp Obstet Gynecol 1997;24(4):228–31.

75. Zarutskie PW, Phillips JA. A meta-analysis of the route of administration of luteal phase support in assisted reproductive technology: vaginal versus intramuscular progesterone. Fertil Steril 2009;92(1):163–9.

76. Miles RA, Paulson RJ, Lobo RA, et al. Pharmacokinetics and endometrial tissue levels of progesterone after administration by intramuscular and vaginal routes: a comparative study. Fertil Steril 1994;62(3):485–90.

77. Mahaguna V, McDermott JM, Zhang F, et al. Investigation of product quality between extemporaneously compounded progesterone vaginal suppositories and an approved progesterone vaginal gel. Drug Dev Ind Pharm 2004;30(10): 1069–78.

78. Doody KJ, Schnell VL, Foulk RA, et al. Endometrin for luteal phase support in a randomized, controlled, open-label, prospective in-vitro fertilization trial using a combination of Menopur and Bravelle for controlled ovarian hyperstimulation. Fertil Steril 2009;91(4):1012–7.

79. Zoppetti G, Puppini N, Pizzutti M, et al. Water soluble progesterone–hydroxy-propyl-β-cyclodextrin complex for injectable formulations. J Incl Phenom Macro-cycl Chem 2007;57(1–4):283–8.

80. Sator M, Radicioni M, Cometti B, et al. Pharmacokinetics and safety profile of a novel progesterone aqueous formulation administered by the s.c. route. Gyne-col Endocrinol 2013;29(3):205–8.

81. Lockwood G, Griesinger G, Cometti B, 13 European Centers. Subcutaneous progesterone versus vaginal progesterone gel for luteal phase support in in vitro fertilization: a noninferiority randomized controlled study. Fertil Steril 2014;101(1):112–9.e3.

82. Baker VL, Jones CA, Doody K, et al. A randomized, controlled trial comparing the efficacy and safety of aqueous subcutaneous progesterone with vaginal progesterone for luteal phase support of in vitro fertilization. Hum Reprod 2014;29:2212–20.

83. Baruffi R, Mauri AL, Petersen CG, et al. Effects of vaginal progesterone admin-istration starting on the day of oocyte retrieval on pregnancy rates. J Assist Re-prod Genet 2003;20(12):517–20.

84. Mochtar MH, Van Wely M, Van der Veen F. Timing luteal phase support in GnRH agonist down-regulated IVF/embryo transfer cycles. Hum Reprod 2006;21(4): 905–8.

85. Prapas Y, Prapas N, Jones EE, et al. The window for embryo transfer in oocyte donation cycles depends on the duration of progesterone therapy. Hum Reprod 1998;13(3):720–3.

86. Liu XR, Mu HQ, Shi Q, et al. The optimal duration of progesterone supplemen-tation in pregnant women after IVF/ICSI: a meta-analysis. Reprod Biol Endocri-nol 2012;10(1):107.

87. Fatemi HM, Popovic-Todorovic B, Papanikolaou E, et al. An update of luteal phase support in stimulated IVF cycles. Hum Reprod Update 2007;13(6):581–90.

88. Kolibianakis EM, Venetis CA, Papanikolaou EG, et al. Estrogen addition to pro-gesterone for luteal phase support in cycles stimulated with GnRH analogues and gonadotrophins for IVF: a systematic review and meta-analysis. Hum Re-prod 2008;23(6):1346–54.

89. Pirard C, Donnez J, Loumaye E. GnRH agonist as novel luteal support: results of a randomized, parallel group, feasibility study using intranasal administration of buserelin. Hum Reprod 2005;20(7):1798–804.

90. Oliveira JB, Baruffi R, Petersen CG, et al. Administration of single-dose GnRH agonist in the luteal phase in ICSI cycles: a meta-analysis. Reprod Biol Endocri-nol 2010;8(1):107.

91. Tesarik J, Hazout A, Mendoza-Tesarik R, et al. Beneficial effect of luteal-phase GnRH agonist administration on embryo implantation after ICSI in both GnRH agonist- and antagonist-treated ovarian stimulation cycles. Hum Reprod 2006; 21(10):2572–9.

92. Ata B, Yakin K, Balaban B, et al. GnRH agonist protocol administration in the luteal phase in ICSI-ET cycles stimulated with the long GnRH agonist protocol: a randomized, controlled double blind study. Hum Reprod 2008;23(3):668–73.

93. Isik AZ, Caglar GS, Sozen E, et al. Single-dose GnRH agonist administration in the luteal phase of GnRH antagonist cycles: a prospective randomized study. Reprod Biomed Online 2009;19(4):472–7.

94. Razieh DF, Maryam AR, Nasim T. Beneficial effect of luteal-phase gonadotropin-releasing hormone agonist administration on implantation rate after intracyto-plasmic sperm injection. Taiwan J Obstet Gynecol 2009;48(3):245–8.

95. Ata B, Urman B. Single dose GnRH agonist administration in the luteal phase of assisted reproduction cycles: is the effect dependent on the type of GnRH analogue used for pituitary suppression? Reprod Biomed Online 2010;20(1): 165–6.
96. Casper RF. Luteal phase support for frozen embryo transfer cycles: intramuscular or vaginal progesterone? Fertil Steril 2014;101(3):627–8.
97. Gibbons WE, Toner JP, Hamacher P, et al. Experience with a novel vaginal progesterone preparation in a donor oocyte program. Fertil Steril 1998;69(1): 96–101.
98. Jobanputra K, Toner JP, Denoncourt R, et al. Crinone 8% (90 mg) given once daily for progesterone replacement therapy in donor egg cycles. Fertil Steril 1999;72(6):980–4.
99. Berger BM, Phillips JA. Pregnancy outcomes in oocyte donation recipients: vaginal gel versus intramuscular injection progesterone replacement. J Assist Reprod Genet 2012;29(3):237–42.
100. Shapiro DB, Pappadakis JA, Ellsworth NM, et al. Progesterone replacement with vaginal gel versus i.m. injection: cycle and pregnancy outcomes in IVF patients receiving vitrified blastocysts. Hum Reprod 2014;29(8):1706–11.
101. Kaser DJ, Ginsburg ES, Missmer SA, et al. Intramuscular progesterone versus 8% Crinone vaginal gel for luteal phase support for day 3 cryopreserved embryo transfer. Fertil Steril 2012;98(6):1464–9.
102. Haddad G, Saguan DA, Maxwell R, et al. Intramuscular route of progesterone administration increases pregnancy rates during non-downregulated frozen embryo transfer cycles. J Assist Reprod Genet 2007;24(10):467–70.
103. Nawroth F, Ludwig M. What is the "ideal" duration of progesterone supplementation before the transfer of cryopreserved-thawed embryos in estrogen/progesterone replacement protocols? Hum Reprod 2005;20(5):1127–34.

Premature Ovarian Failure

Clinical Presentation and Treatment

Ertug Kovanci, MD*, Amy K. Schutt, MD

KEYWORDS

- Infertility • Estrogen therapy • Ovarian failure • Autoimmune disorders
- Heart disease • Osteoporosis

KEY POINTS

- Long-term health consequences, including psychological distress, infertility, osteoporosis, heart disease, autoimmune disorders, and increased mortality, have a significant impact on the quality of life for the woman diagnosed with premature ovarian failure.
- Initiation of hormone replacement therapy (HRT) should be initiated immediately without considering the Women's Health Initiative findings.
- Donor oocyte in vitro fertilization has high pregnancy rates.

INTRODUCTION AND TERMINOLOGY

Premature ovarian failure (POF) is defined as hypergonadotropic hypogonadism with the cessation of menses before age 40. About 1% to 3% of women experience POF before age 40.[1,2] The incidence is lower in younger women. A follicle stimulating hormone (FSH) concentration greater than 20 to 40 mIU/mL in the presence of amenorrhea has been proposed to define ovarian failure.[3] The presumption of ovarian failure is evidenced by the association between decreased natural fecundity and lowered assisted reproductive technology success rates with increased FSH concentrations and increased age. When the FSH concentrations are greater than 12 to 15 mIU/mL in women who are less than the age of 40 years with regular cycles, the ovaries are unlikely to respond to the stimulating agents, such as human menopausal gonadotropins and recombinant FSH. On the other hand, some women who are diagnosed with POF may become pregnant spontaneously albeit the likelihood is low. Therefore, the term "primary ovarian insufficiency" has been proposed as an alternative to POF by some investigators.[4,5] This new term sounds like it covers different spectrums of the disorder and, thus, may be more appropriate for clinical use. However, the term

Authors have no conflict of interests to disclose.
Division of Reproductive Endocrinology and Infertility, Department of Obstetrics and Gynecology, Baylor College of Medicine, 6651 Main Street, Suite F350, Houston, TX 77030, USA
* Corresponding author.
E-mail address: ekovanci@bcm.edu

Obstet Gynecol Clin N Am 42 (2015) 153–161
http://dx.doi.org/10.1016/j.ogc.2014.10.004
0889-8545/15/$ – see front matter © 2015 Elsevier Inc. All rights reserved.

primary ovarian insufficiency may lead to phenotypic heterogeneity in translational studies. Recruitment of heterogeneous study populations may prevent finding significant associations between the disorder and the genotype. Even the current term POF includes a heterogeneous group of women as the various clinical presentations suggest. Manifestations of POF, defined as an FSH level greater than 40 mIU/mL with amenorrhea before age 40, include primary amenorrhea, secondary amenorrhea, presence or absence of autoimmune disorders, and association with chromosomal abnormalities such as Turner syndrome, all of which imply different causes. Moreover, the authors do not think insufficiency has a better connotation than failure, and these 2 words are actually synonyms. To prevent unnecessary confusion in the literature, the continued use of the term POF is suggested.

CAUSE

It is well known that X chromosome abnormalities are the underlying cause in some cases of POF. The most common of these abnormalities is 45,X or Turner syndrome, which affects 1 in 2500 female newborns worldwide.[6] It is thought that 75% or more of conceptions affected by Turner syndrome result in spontaneous abortion.[7] Turner syndrome is characterized clinically by short stature, cardiovascular anomalies (especially coarctation of the aorta and aortic valvular abnormalities), webbed neck, lymphedema, and POF.

In addition to Turner syndrome, other X chromosome aberrations, such as deletions of the short or long arm of the X chromosome, have been shown to be associated with POF.[6] These deletions show variable phenotype depending on the location of the deletion. Proximal deletions of Xq are associated with primary amenorrhea especially if these originate more proximal than Xq21.[6] Similarly, the amount of remaining Xp also affects the phenotype.[6] The numerous cases of X chromosome abnormalities and POF have led to the identification of a "critical region" at Xq13.3-Xq27. Several candidate genes in this region have been suggested; however, the exact contributors remain elusive.

Autosomal chromosomal abnormalities and balanced autosomal reciprocal translocations can also be associated with POF. Necropsy examinations on fetuses with trisomy 13 and 18 revealed findings consistent with ovarian dysgenesis.[8] Numerous autosomal genes are known to affect ovarian development, and translocations involving a sex chromosome and autosome may affect autosomal gene expression, and/or meiosis I progression.[8]

POF can also be part of various phenotypic abnormalities that are seen in well-defined Mendelian disorders. Autoimmune polyendocrine syndrome (APS) type 1 and 2 show multiple endocrine organ failures including adrenal insufficiency, hypoparathyroidism, hypothyroidism, type 1 diabetes mellitus, and ovarian failure. APS type 1 is caused by mutations in the AIRE gene.[9] Perrault syndrome is an autosomal-recessive disorder involving POF and neurosensory deafness. The connexin 37 gene is an attractive candidate for this disorder because the connexin gene family is responsible for many congenital forms of deafness, and the null mice for connexin 37 develop ovarian failure.[10] Another Mendelian disorder associated with POF is ataxia telangiectasia. It involves cerebellar ataxia, telangiectesias, immunodeficiency, genomic instability, and malignancy.[11] The gene that has been found to be mutated in patients with ataxi-telangiectasia is named the ATM gene.[12] Women with type I blepharophimosis, ptosis, epicanthus inversus syndrome can present with POF.[13] FOXL2 mutations have been identified in these women. Fragile X syndrome is of note because not only does it have an intricate genetic origin but also it is one of the most common causes of POF. Fragile X premutation carriers are at risk for POF; however, women with the full mutation are not at risk. The incidence of fragile X premutations (carrier state) in women with POF was found to be between 3% and 12% depending on the family history.[14] On the other hand, approximately 20% of the fragile X carriers develop POF.[15]

More than 100 mouse models involving gonosomal or autosomal genes exhibit ovarian failure.[8] Best known models include growth differentiating factor 9, newborn ovary homeobox, G protein-coupled receptor, and factor in germline α knock-out animals, all preferentially expressed in the oocytes.

Perturbations of somatic genes can also cause POF because these genes are involved in human ovarian development and function. Examples include follicle stimulating hormone receptor (*FSHR*) and luteinizing hormone receptor (*LHR*).

In summary, a large group of candidate genes for idiopathic POF have been derived based on the genes that are deleted or located in the autosomal or sex chromosomal breakpoints, animal models of ovarian failure, genes involved in syndromic POF cases, and genes involved in ovarian development and function. However, studies that investigated the perturbations of candidate genes in women with idiopathic POF in different ethnic populations yielded no association or weak associations with low incidence. It is estimated that the cause of 90% of the primary POF cases still remains unknown.[16] It is clear that POF is a genetically highly heterogeneous disorder, because mouse knockouts in more than 100 different genes prematurely lose ovarian function. These results likely explain the low yields observed in clinical studies with single candidate gene approaches.

Recently, genome-wide association studies (GWAS) have focused on age at menopause and POF. GWAS were aimed at finding associations between genotype markers and phenotype in very large patient and control populations. Several GWAS have been conducted in various ethnic populations to identify the genotypes associated with age at menopause and POF.[17–19] The quest to identify the genetic mutation leading to POF continues.

DIAGNOSTIC WORKUP

Diagnostic workup is usually triggered by the absence of menarche, the cessation of menses, or infertility. Clinical presentation dictates the type of workup necessary (**Box 1**). A physical examination to rule out other reproductive disorders is indicated. It should include a thorough general and pelvic examination, including the breast, axillary hair, and pubic hair development. A pelvic ultrasound may be necessary if an adequate pelvic examination cannot be performed. Primary amenorrhea can be caused by various congenital disorders, such as Mullerian agenesis, androgen insensitivity, and XY gonadal dysgenesis or Swyer syndrome. However, the most common

Box 1
Most commonly performed initial workup
Serum FSH
Karyotype
Fragile X carrier screening
Serum TSH
Dual energy x-ray absorptiometry scan

reason for primary amenorrhea with hypergonadotropic hypogonadism is 45,X, or Turner syndrome. All women with primary amenorrhea should undergo serum FSH measurement. If the FSH level is found to be elevated, karyotyping is indicated to determine if Turner syndrome or a rare male pseudohermaphroditism syndrome is present. Karyotyping also allows the identification of other chromosomal aberrations such as X chromosome deletions and autosomal translocations.

Secondary amenorrhea should prompt urinary or serum pregnancy testing. After an unexpected pregnancy is ruled out, prolactin and thyroid stimulating hormone (TSH) levels should be determined to exclude hyperprolactinemia and thyroid disorders, which frequently cause menstrual abnormalities. If prolactin and TSH levels are within normal limits, progestin challenge test is performed to produce withdrawal bleeding. In the absence of withdrawal bleeding, which indicates hypoestrogenism or a reproductive tract outlet problem, the FSH level should be determined. Alternatively, an FSH level may be included in the initial workup if clinically indicated based on the presentation. Classically, 2 FSH levels greater than 40 mIU/mL, performed 1 month apart, indicate POF. More recently, an anti-Müllerian hormone (AMH) concentration less than 1.0 ng/mL has been shown to reflect a diminished ovarian reserve. However, this should not be confused with POF because even women with undetectable AMH levels frequently continue to have regular periods and FSH concentrations less than 15 mIU/mL. A high FSH level continues to be the preferred diagnostic test. On the other hand, very low levels of AMH may be the first sign of impending POF and could be used as an early screening test. More research is needed to determine the predictive value of very low AMH levels.

Once the POF diagnosis is established, karyotyping may be performed to rule out structural autosomal and sex chromosomal abnormalities as well as Turner syndrome and mosaic Turner syndrome (45,X/46,XX). Many experts suggest checking the karyotype in women who are younger and have never been pregnant. The value of chromosome analysis is diminished in women who are older than 30 to 35 years old and have had a child. On the other hand, fragile X carrier screening is recommended to all women with POF by the American College of Obstetricians and Gynecologists.[20] The CGG repeat numbers between 55 and 200 in the FMR gene increase the risk for POF.[20]

CLINICAL PICTURE

The diagnosis of POF can be devastating for patients. POF is a disorder that will have long-term effects on reproductive capabilities as well as on general health (**Box 2**). Women with POF report more anxiety, depression, and psychological distress than

---

Box 2
Long-term consequences of premature ovarian failure

Infertility

Psychological distress and depression

Decreased sexual and general well-being

Autoimmune disorders

Osteoporosis

Ischemic heart disease

Increased risk for mortality

controls.[21] Therefore, supportive therapy and psychological counseling may be helpful, but is overlooked frequently.

Clinical consequences of hypoestrogenemia such as osteoporosis and genital atrophy may have a significant impact on the quality of life. Bone mass loss develops rapidly after ovarian failure. Vaginal atrophy manifests with dryness, irritation, and dyspareunia. Coupled with emotional distress because of fertility concerns, genital atrophy may easily strain the patient's personal life. Women with POF are less satisfied with their sexual lives and complain more frequently about diminished general and sexual well-being than controls.[21] Their androgen concentrations are also decreased significantly, which contributed to sexual dysfunction.

Various autoimmune disorders are associated with POF. Autoimmune hypothyroidism, adrenal insufficiency, type 1 diabetes mellitus, pernicious anemia, and hypoparathyroidism have been reported in the literature (**Box 3**). Hypothyroidism is the most common autoimmune disorder in association with POF. The incidence of hypothyroidism in women with POF is about 8%.[22] Other autoimmune disorders are relatively uncommon. The incidence of diabetes mellitus has been shown to be 2.5%. Although clinically symptomatic adrenal insufficiency is rare, it has been reported that 3.2% of women with POF have adrenal antibodies to the 21-hydroxylase enzyme.[22]

Future pregnancy with autologous oocytes is considered impossible in women with primary amenorrhea and Turner syndrome. On the other hand, about 5% to 10% of women with secondary amenorrhea and hypergonadotropic hypogonadism may ovulate spontaneously and become pregnant. However, most women with POF have a low likelihood of a spontaneous pregnancy. It is almost impossible to predict which women will ovulate and become pregnant. The only successful fertility treatment option is in vitro fertilization (IVF) using donated oocytes. Women with Turner syndrome are not recommended to become pregnant even with donor oocytes because of the high rates of mortality during pregnancy resulting from aortic aneurysm rupture. It has been shown that the risk of aortic aneurysm rupture cannot be determined based on the size of the aortic root dilatation.[23] Pregnancy should be avoided in Turner syndrome.

Observational studies suggest cardiovascular disease risk is increased in women with POF.[24] A secondary analysis of the Danish Nurse Cohort study reported a 2.1-fold increased risk for ischemic heart disease in women who experienced menopause before age 40 compared women with age of menopause greater than 45.[25] Hormone replacement therapy (HRT) decreased this risk in women whose POF was due to the surgical removal of bilateral ovaries. This increased risk may be partly due to impaired endothelial function, which can also be reversed with HRT.[26]

Box 3
Autoimmune diseases associated with premature ovarian failure

Hypothyroidism

Adrenal insufficiency

Type 1 diabetes mellitus

Pernicious anemia

Hypoparathyroidism

Myasthenia gravis

Rheumatoid arthritis

Systemic lupus erythematosus

Overall mortality was also found to be increased in women with POF.[27] A Norwegian study including about 20,000 women with a 37-year follow-up showed that women who had menopause before age 40 experienced the highest rates of mortality.[2] Ischemic heart disease, stroke, and cancers were the most common causes for mortality in this study.

MANAGEMENT

Prevention of consequences of hypoestrogenemia must be the first goal of the management. These women should be offered HRT as soon as POF is diagnosed. The form of HRT can be selected based on the patient's preference. HRT regiments that are used in postmenopausal women can be considered. However, women with POF may require higher doses of estrogen than postmenopausal women. Oral contraceptives (OCPs) present a good alternative to postmenopausal HRT regiments. OCPs generally have 2-fold to 4-fold higher estrogen content than postmenopausal HRT regiments. Another benefit of OCPs is that many of the peers of these patients will be taking OCPs for birth control, possibly increasing patients' satisfaction with the treatment. The counseling regarding the risks of the HRT in these patients should be similar to the counseling of other reproductive-aged women who are interested in hormonal contraception. The findings of the Women's Health Initiative (WHI) study, such as increased risk for breast cancer, heart attack, and stroke, should not be considered relevant to these women. It is important to remember that none of the postmenopausal HRT studies included women who were younger than the age of 40.[28,29] The average age was 63 in both arms of the WHI study. If women with POF consider staying on HRT after age 50, then they can be counseled appropriately based on the findings of the WHI and other similar studies in postmenopausal women. The route of the estrogen therapy, on the other hand, may affect the side-effect profile. For patients who are at risk for thromboembolic events such as smokers, the transdermal route may be preferred. The ESTHER study demonstrated that the transdermal estrogen therapy does not increase the risk of deep venous thrombosis (DVT).[30] The same study also showed that certain types of progestins can increase the DVT risk, whereas progesterone has no effect on the DVT risk. Furthermore, the transdermal estrogen therapy in postmenopausal women did not increase the stroke risk in the British nested stroke study.[31] Taken together, all these studies suggest transdermal estrogen therapy combined with oral micronized progesterone may have a better side-effect profile than oral estrogens combined with progestins. The authors' preferred estrogen therapy regiment in women who are not interested in taking OCPs is transdermal estrogen patch or cream combined with cyclical oral micronized progesterone every 1 to 3 months.

Topical estrogen supplementation should be used in women with POF who continue to have vaginal complaints despite the systemic HRT. Vaginal atrophy may be a continued concern even on systemic therapy in women with primary amenorrhea. A topical approach is also an excellent option for progesterone supplementation because vaginal progesterone cream and pills are easily absorbed and yield very high tissue levels in the uterus. It has been estimated the tissue levels of progesterone are 4 times higher compared with intramuscular or oral use. Vaginal progesterone pills are less messy compared with the cream. Thus, it is preferred for HRT in women with POF. However, the cost can be a problem for vaginal progesterone medications. A new oral medication, ospimefene, is a selective estrogen receptor modulator with estrogenic effects on the vaginal mucosa in clinical studies and antiestrogenic effects on the breast in animal studies.[32,33] Ospimefene can be considered for women with dyspareunia due to atrophic changes of the vagina if patients are adverse to vaginal treatments.

Osteoporosis is serious concern as the maximum bone density is reached in the mid-twenties. Prompt diagnosis and treatment are crucial to achieve the maximum bone health. Bone density measurement should be considered, especially for women whose diagnosis was delayed, thus, who did not receive HRT for a long period of time. Calcium and vitamin D supplementation is recommended. Daily requirement for Calcium is 1000 to 1500 mg for reproductive-aged women, most of which can be obtained through diet if encouraged. Many women are found to have low vitamin D levels in today's society. The authors recommend routinely checking vitamin D levels. Recommended daily supplementation dose for postmenopausal women is 800 IU. However, if the vitamin D levels are found to be low, high doses up to 50,000 units weekly can be administered. If osteoporosis is detected, an antiresorptive therapy such as bisphosphonates should be considered in women who are already on estrogen therapy. There are newer antiresorptive therapies such Denosumab. Alendronate, Risedronate, Zoledronic acid, and Denosumab are considered first-line therapy.[34] Ibandronate is a second-line agent, and Raloxifene is considered a second-line or third-line agent. Teriparatide, a parathyroid hormone analogue, is recommended for patients with very high fracture risk or for failed bisphosphonate therapy. Calcitonin should be used as the last line of therapy. However, most of the data and recommendations are for postmenopausal women, which are not as robust for younger women with POF. Data from premenopausal women with osteoporosis due to other chronic medical problems such as systemic lupus erythematosus, cystic fibrosis, or chronic kidney disease suggest medical treatment with various agents may be beneficial.

Screening for other autoimmune disorders seems to be prudent. TSH is probably the single most important test for this purpose. Fasting blood glucose, complete blood count, serum calcium, and adrenal antibodies to the 21-hydroxylase enzyme may be helpful in the identification of other autoimmune disorders. The authors routinely screen for TSH abnormalities and selectively screen for other autoimmune disorders based on presentation after taking a careful history and physical examination. Measurement of antiovarian antibodies is not helpful because they have no clinical meaning nor do they change the management. Thus, it is not recommended to obtain antiovarian antibody levels.

Various clinical studies failed to show significant benefit from various fertility treatments such estrogen priming followed by IVF except for occasional case reports. Ovarian biopsy via laparoscopy or transvaginal ultrasound examinations to determine follicular activity has not been shown to correlate with pregnancy or infertility treatment success. Therefore, routine clinical use of these methods is not recommended. Estrogen pretreatment and various ovarian stimulation protocols involving high-dose gonadotropins or different down-regulation methods proved to be fruitless. On the other hand, IVF using donated oocytes has very high pregnancy rates. It also allows for the genetic contribution of the patient's partner and for the patient to experience pregnancy and childbirth. Women with POF should be counseled regarding availability of donor oocyte IVF. However, Turner syndrome is considered a contraindication to pregnancy. Gestational carrier receiving embryos formed with donor oocytes and partner's sperm is an option for women with Turner syndrome.

In summary, POF is a devastating diagnosis that has significant emotional and clinical long-term consequences. Timely diagnosis, counseling, and intervention may alleviate some of these consequences.

REFERENCES

1. Coulam CB, Adamson SC, Annegers JF. Incidence of premature ovarian failure. Obstet Gynecol 1986;67(4):604–6.
2. Jacobsen BK, Heuch I, Kvale G. Age at natural menopause and all-cause mortality: a 37-year follow-up of 19,731 Norwegian women. Am J Epidemiol 2003;157(10): 923–9.
3. Kovanci E, Rohozinski J, Simpson JL, et al. Growth differentiating factor-9 mutations may be associated with premature ovarian failure. Fertil Steril 2007;87(1):143–6.
4. Simpson JL. Genetic and phenotypic heterogeneity in ovarian failure: overview of selected candidate genes. Ann N Y Acad Sci 2008;1135:146–54.
5. Welt CK. Primary ovarian insufficiency: a more accurate term for premature ovarian failure. Clin Endocrinol (Oxf) 2008;68(4):499–509.
6. Simpson JL, Elias S. Genetics in obstetrics and gynecology. 3rd edition. Philadelphia: Saunders; 2003.
7. Hook EB, Warburton D. The distribution of chromosomal genotypes associated with Turner's syndrome: livebirth prevalence rates and evidence for diminished fetal mortality and severity in genotypes associated with structural X abnormalities or mosaicism. Hum Genet 1983;64(1):24–7.
8. Simpson JL, Rajkovic A. Ovarian differentiation and gonadal failure. Am J Med Genet 1999;89(4):186–200.
9. Wolff AS, Erichsen MM, Meager A, et al. Autoimmune polyendocrine syndrome type 1 in Norway: phenotypic variation, autoantibodies, and novel mutations in the autoimmune regulator gene. J Clin Endocrinol Metab 2007;92(2):595–603.
10. Simon AM, Goodenough DA, Li E, et al. Female infertility in mice lacking connexin 37. Nature 1997;385(6616):525–9.
11. Dunn HG, Meuwissen H, Livingstone CS, et al. Ataxia-telangiectasia. Can Med Assoc J 1964;91:1106–18.
12. McKinnon PJ. ATM and the molecular pathogenesis of ataxia telangiectasia. Annu Rev Pathol 2012;7:303–21.
13. De Baere E, Dixon MJ, Small KW, et al. Spectrum of FOXL2 gene mutations in blepharophimosis-ptosis-epicanthus inversus (BPES) families demonstrates a genotype–phenotype correlation. Hum Mol Genet 2001;10(15):1591–600.
14. Sherman SL. Premature ovarian failure in the fragile X syndrome. Am J Med Genet 2000;97(3):189–94.
15. Ennis S, Ward D, Murray A. Nonlinear association between CGG repeat number and age of menopause in FMR1 premutation carriers. Eur J Hum Genet 2006; 14(2):253–5.
16. Nelson LM. Clinical practice. Primary ovarian insufficiency. N Engl J Med 2009; 360(6):606–14.
17. He C, Kraft P, Chen C, et al. Genome-wide association studies identify loci associated with age at menarche and age at natural menopause. Nat Genet 2009; 41(6):724–8.
18. Knauff EA, Franke L, van Es MA, et al. Genome-wide association study in premature ovarian failure patients suggests ADAMTS19 as a possible candidate gene. Hum Reprod 2009;24(9):2372–8.
19. Perry JR, Corre T, Esko T, et al. A genome-wide association study of early menopause and the combined impact of identified variants. Hum Mol Genet 2013; 22(7):1465–72.
20. American College of Obstetricians and Gynecologists. ACOG Committee opinion no. 469: carrier screening for fragile X syndrome. Obstet Gynecol 2010;116(4):1008–10.

21. van der Stege JG, Groen H, van Zadelhoff SJ, et al. Decreased androgen concentrations and diminished general and sexual well-being in women with premature ovarian failure. Menopause 2008;15(1):23–31.
22. Takebayashi K, Takakura K, Wang H, et al. Mutation analysis of the growth differentiation factor-9 and -9B genes in patients with premature ovarian failure and polycystic ovary syndrome. Fertil Steril 2000;74(5):976–9.
23. Karnis MF. Fertility, pregnancy, and medical management of Turner syndrome in the reproductive years. Fertil Steril 2012;98(4):787–91.
24. Atsma F, Bartelink ML, Grobbee DE, et al. Postmenopausal status and early menopause as independent risk factors for cardiovascular disease: a meta-analysis. Menopause 2006;13(2):265–79.
25. Lokkegaard E, Jovanovic Z, Heitmann BL, et al. The association between early menopause and risk of ischaemic heart disease: influence of Hormone Therapy. Maturitas 2006;53(2):226–33.
26. Kalantaridou SN, Naka KK, Papanikolaou E, et al. Impaired endothelial function in young women with premature ovarian failure: normalization with hormone therapy. J Clin Endocrinol Metab 2004;89(8):3907–13.
27. Mondul AM, Rodriguez C, Jacobs EJ, et al. Age at natural menopause and cause-specific mortality. Am J Epidemiol 2005;162(11):1089–97.
28. Anderson GL, Limacher M, Assaf AR, et al. Effects of conjugated equine estrogen in postmenopausal women with hysterectomy: the Women's Health Initiative randomized controlled trial. JAMA 2004;291(14):1701–12.
29. Rossouw JE, Anderson GL, Prentice RL, et al. Risks and benefits of estrogen plus progestin in healthy postmenopausal women: principal results From the Women's Health Initiative randomized controlled trial. JAMA 2002;288(3):321–33.
30. Canonico M, Oger E, Plu-Bureau G, et al. Hormone therapy and venous thromboembolism among postmenopausal women: impact of the route of estrogen administration and progestogens: the ESTHER study. Circulation 2007;115(7): 840–5.
31. Renoux C, Dell'aniello S, Garbe E, et al. Transdermal and oral hormone replacement therapy and the risk of stroke: a nested case-control study. BMJ 2010;340: c2519.
32. Bachmann GA, Komi JO, Ospemifene Study Group. Ospemifene effectively treats vulvovaginal atrophy in postmenopausal women: results from a pivotal phase 3 study. Menopause 2010;17(3):480–6.
33. Kangas L, Unkila M. Tissue selectivity of ospemifene: pharmacologic profile and clinical implications. Steroids 2013;78(12–13):1273–80.
34. Khan SN, Craig L, Wild R. Osteoporosis: therapeutic guidelines. Guidelines for practice management of osteoporosis. Clin Obstet Gynecol 2013;56(4): 694–702.

Hormonal and Nonhormonal Treatment of Vasomotor Symptoms

Miriam S. Krause, MD[a],*, Steven T. Nakajima, MD[b]

KEYWORDS

- Menopause • Vasomotor symptoms • Estrogen • Progestogen • SSRI • SNRI

KEY POINTS

- Hot flashes are the most common complaint of perimenopause.
- Treatment has to be individualized based on the risk/benefit ratio.
- Systemic hormone therapy is the most effective treatment.
- Nonhormonal pharmacologic therapies include selective serotonin reuptake inhibitors, selective norepinephrine reuptake inhibitors, clonidine, and gabapentin.
- Nonpharmacologic therapies are considered less effective and include behavioral changes and possibly acupuncture.

GENERAL HEALTH MAINTENANCE AND CARE OF MENOPAUSAL WOMEN

The American College of Obstetricians and Gynecologists (ACOG) recommends an annual history and physical examination including breast and pelvic examination. **Box 1** lists guidelines specifically for the health maintenance and care of perimenopausal and postmenopausal women. **Table 1** summarizes terms helpful in describing menopausal events.

HOT FLASHES/VASOMOTOR SYMPTOMS
What Are Hot Flashes?

Hot flashes and hot flushes can be used as synonyms. If they occur at night, they are often called night sweats. They are characterized by the sudden onset of heat, intense sweating, and flushing of the face and chest, often accompanied by palpitations and

Financial Disclosures: S.T. Nakajima was a member of the Speakers Bureau of Noven Therapeutics, LLC. M.S. Krause has no financial disclosures.
[a] Fertility and Endocrine Associates, 4121 Dutchman's Lane, Suite 414, Louisville, KY 40207, USA; [b] Stanford Fertility and Reproductive Medicine Center, 900 Welch Road, Suite 20, Palo Alto, CA 94304, USA
* Corresponding author.
E-mail address: ms.krause@yahoo.de

Obstet Gynecol Clin N Am 42 (2015) 163–179
http://dx.doi.org/10.1016/j.ogc.2014.09.008
0889-8545/15/$ – see front matter © 2015 Elsevier Inc. All rights reserved.

obgyn.theclinics.com

Box 1
Health care of perimenopausal and postmenopausal women

Evaluate sexuality, fitness, psychosocial factors, cardiovascular factors, and health risk behaviors annually

Physical examination including breast and pelvic examination annually

Pap test (per ACOG guidelines, can be discontinued at age 65 years after 3 consecutive negative cytology results or 2 consecutive negative cotest results (cytology and HPV) within the previous 10 years, and the most recent test no longer than 5 years ago, and no history of CIN2 or CIN3)

Mammogram every 1 to 2 years between the ages of 40 and 50 years, then yearly

Colonoscopy every 10 years starting at age 50 years (age 45 years for African American patients) unless risk factors present (other screening options available but not preferred)

Fasting glucose every 3 years starting at age 45 years

Fasting lipid panel every 5 years starting at age 45 years

Thyroid-stimulating hormone every 5 years starting at age 50 years

Aspirin prophylaxis at age 55 to 79 years if no contraindications (and no concern for gastrointestinal bleeding)

Herpes zoster vaccine once at age 60 years, if not previously immunized

DEXA (starting at age 65 years unless risk factors, repeat no sooner than after 2 years)

Pneumococcal vaccine once at age 65 years

HCV testing (once if born between 1945 and 1965 and not yet assessed)

HIV testing (offer annually based on risk factors)

Influenza vaccine annually

TDaP (substitute 1 dose of TDaP with TD, followed by booster every 10 years)

Varicella vaccine (1 series if no evidence of immunity)

Abbreviations: CIN, cervical intraepithelial neoplasia; DEXA, dual-energy x-ray absorptiometry; HCV, hepatitis C virus; HIV, human immunodeficiency virus; HPV, human papilloma virus; TD, tetanus diphtheria; TDaP, tetanus diphtheria acellular pertussis.

Additional recommendations exist for high risk patients. For more details, visit www.acog.org/~/media/Departments/Annual Womens Health Care/PrimaryAndPreventiveCare.pdf.

---

anxiety.[1] Hot flashes are considered the cardinal symptom of menopause[1] and, although they cause no inherent health hazard, they are the most bothersome symptom caused by estrogen withdrawal for most women. Therefore, they are clinically relevant in the everyday gynecologic practice. Furthermore, vasomotor symptoms

Table 1
Menopausal terms

Term (WHO)	Definition
Perimenopause	Time period with a break in regular menstrual cycles with the break lasting no longer than 3 mo
Late perimenopause	Amenorrhea between 4 and 11 mo
Menopause	Amenorrhea for 12 mo or longer Median age in the United States: 51 y

Abbreviation: WHO, World Health Organization.

are among the clear indications for US Food and Drug Administration (FDA)–approved hormone therapy.

Cause of hot flashes

The cause of hot flashes is not well understood and most likely multifactorial. The menopausal transition coincides with declining estrogen levels, and treatment with estrogen improves or even relieves vasomotor symptoms. The decline in estrogen levels seems more relevant than the absolute estrogen levels.[2] Women who have never been exposed to estrogens, such as women with Turner syndrome, do not report hot flashes because of the absence of estrogen priming, because these women are hypogonadal at birth. During the perimenopause, the ratio of specific types of estrogens changes: estradiol levels decrease and levels of estrone, a weaker estrogen, increase.[3]

In addition, beginning with the perimenopause, narrowing of the thermoneutral zone occurs[4]: The thermoneutral zone describes a homeostatic range of body temperature. Sweating occurs when the body core temperature increases above the upper threshold of the thermoneutral zone, and chills occur with dipping of the core temperature below the lower threshold. A smaller thermoneutral zone leads to greater likelihood of crossing both the upper and lower thresholds, and therefore puts a woman at higher propensity for developing sweating and chills.[4] Neurotransmitters are involved in the regulation of the thermoneutral zone: as estrogen levels decline, norepinephrine levels increase, which causes an increase in hypothalamic serotonin receptors, and further narrowing of the thermoneutral zone.[5–7] The exact mechanism of action of selective serotonin reuptake inhibitors (SSRIs) on the improvement of hot flashes is unknown but seems to be related to this. In theory, the increase in the number of serotonin receptors leads to a decrease in circulating serotonin levels in the brain. When women use SSRIs, levels of serotonin increase within the brain, with an expected widening of the thermoneutral zone and, as a consequence, improvement in vasomotor symptoms.

Estrogen depletion also stimulates central alpha-2 receptors, which causes a further increase in norepinephrine levels and, as a consequence, further narrowing of the thermoneutral zone (**Fig. 1**).

Risk factors for hot flashes

African American women are most likely to report vasomotor symptoms, whereas Chinese and Japanese women are the least likely. Women of different ethnic backgrounds show genetic polymorphisms for the estrogen receptor alpha and enzymes involved in the sex-steroid pathways. These polymorphisms can have an effect on estrogen metabolism, circulating estrogen concentration, and severity of vasomotor symptoms.[8]

Obesity was originally thought to be protective secondary to the higher conversion of androgens to estrogens in the adipose tissue, but this has not proved correct. Adipose tissue acts as a heat insulator and can make hot flashes worse.

Nicotine is another risk factor. Women who smoke enter menopause on average 2 to 3 years earlier than nonsmokers, and have a 60% higher risk for hot flashes because of the antiestrogenic effects of nicotine.

Negative mood and affect and a history of child abuse or neglect are also risk factors, possibly because of a lack of coping skills when presented with social and lifestyle stress. Lower socioeconomic position may either present a true risk factor or be a confounder. Lower socioeconomic position is associated with smoking, higher body mass index, and higher stress levels, which are all risk factors for more vasomotor symptoms.[1]

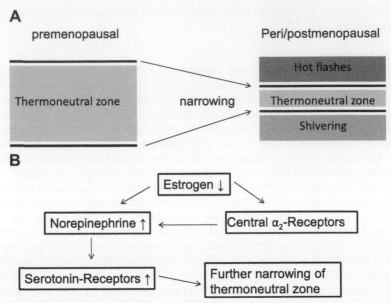

Fig. 1. Thermoneutral zone (*A*) and involved neurotransmitter (*B*). (*Modified from* [*A*] Pachman DR, Jones JM, Loprinzi CL. Management of menopause-associated vasomotor symptoms: current treatment options, challenges and future directions. Int J Womens Health 2010;2:123–35; and [*B*] Refs.[5–7])

How Do Hot Flashes Affect Women?

The Study on Women's Health Across the Nation (SWAN), one of the largest and most ethnically diverse longitudinal studies of the perimenopausal transition, enrolled 3302 midlife women across 5 racial/ethnic groups and followed these for more than 10 years, with yearly assessment of menopause-related symptoms, health behaviors, and social/psychological functioning. The SWAN study showed the following results: hot flashes are most common in postmenopausal women (50%–85%), and least common in premenopausal women (20%–40%). In general, 15% to 20% of women report daily flashes. The usual duration of vasomotor symptoms is 1 to 10 years on average, but some women experience them for up to 30 years. This wide range in frequency is thought to be related to different cross-cultural perceptions, which can lead to underreporting as well as overreporting.

Vasomotor symptoms affect sleep quality and quantity. Sleep disorders are subjective and therefore difficult to measure. Per the SWAN study, perimenopausal sleep disorders are most common in white women (40.3%) and least common in Japanese women (28.2%). Sleep disturbances occur even in the absence of vasomotor symptoms, so estrogen withdrawal is not the only factor to blame. Confounding factors include depressed mood, anxiety, back aches, joint pain, low income and financial worries, as well as marital discord, all of which can cause problems sleeping.

Differential diagnoses of hot flashes

In premenopausal women, in whom vasomotor symptoms are the least common, other causes for vasomotor instability have to be considered. Differential diagnoses, and tests to consider after a thorough history and physical examination, are listed in **Table 2**.

Table 2	
Differential diagnoses of hot flashes and tests to order	
Differential Disease State	**Diagnostic Test**
Thyroid disease	Thyroid-stimulating hormone
Subacute/chronic infection	Complete blood count, C-reactive protein
Psychosomatic disorder and stress	Stress questionnaire (eg, Patient Stress Questionnaire)
Leukemia	Complete blood count
Pheochromocytoma	Urine vanillylmandelic acid
Carcinoid	Chromogranin A, urine 5-hydroxy indole acetic acid
Other malignancies	CT or MRI

Abbreviation: CT, computed tomography.

Estrogen (Plus Progestogen) Therapy

Several updates have been published since the controversial Women's Health Initiative (WHI) publication in 2002 reported an association between hormone therapy and breast cancer as well as cardiovascular events. Many of the WHI participants were older women, asymptomatic with regard to hot flashes, postmenopausal when starting hormone therapy, and had significant comorbidities. These characteristics are in contrast with the young, healthy perimenopausal women requesting hormone therapy for hot flashes.

Estrogen therapy

Estrogen therapy is considered the most effective therapy for hot flashes. Guidelines have been published by ACOG, the North American Menopause Society (NAMS), the United States Preventative Services Task Force (USPSTF) and the American Association of Clinical Endocrinologists (AACE). The recommendation is to use "the lowest effective dose for the shortest duration possible in women for whom the potential benefits outweigh the potential risks."

Risks and benefits of estrogen therapy are listed in **Table 3**, with contraindications in **Table 4**. **Table 5** lists the different estrogen formulations with starting doses and routes of administration. Patients should be started on the lowest dose possible, with an increase in the dose if no improvement in symptoms is noted.

The transdermal route should be considered to avoid the hepatic first-pass effect and possibly decrease the risk for venous thromboembolism.[9,10] Lower doses usually require longer duration of treatment until the maximal benefit for vasomotor symptoms is reached. The ultralow dose of estrogen therapy is not FDA approved for the treatment of vasomotor symptoms.

Table 3	
Benefits and risks of hormone therapy initiated during perimenopause	
Benefits	**Future Potential Risks**
Improvement of vasomotor symptoms	Breast cancer
Improvement of vaginal dryness	Cerebrovascular accident (age dependent)
Decreased risk for osteoporosis	Venous thromboembolic event
Decreased risk for colorectal cancer	Possible risk for epithelial ovarian cancer if used longer than 10 y[10,53]

Table 4 Contraindications to using hormone therapy	
Absolute Contraindications	**Relative Contraindications**
Current, past, or suspected breast cancer	Smoking (cigarettes, marijuana)
Known or suspected estrogen-sensitive malignant conditions	
Untreated endometrial hyperplasia	
Undiagnosed vaginal bleeding	
Active liver disease	
Uncontrolled hypertension	
Thrombophilia	
Previous idiopathic or current venous thromboembolism (transdermal application may be acceptable)	
Active or recent arterial thromboembolic event (eg, myocardial infarction)	
Hypersensitivity to any ingredient of the formulation	
Porphyria cutanea tarda	

In assessing the effectiveness of the hormone therapy, it is important for the health care provider to understand that any kind of treatment, hormonal as well as nonhormonal, has a placebo response of up to 51%.[11]

A new FDA-approved hormone combination contains 0.625 mg of conjugated estrogen as well as bazedoxifene 20 mg daily. Bazedoxifene is a selective estrogen receptor modulator (SERM) with antagonistic effects on the endometrium, thereby eliminating the need for additional progestogen therapy.[12] Side effects include muscle spasm, nausea, and diarrhea.

Progestogen therapy

Progestogen therapy is necessary for endometrial protection if a uterus is present, or a possible necessity if the patient has a history of endometriosis. In contrast, progestogens act as mitogens and can cause stimulation of epithelial breast cells.[13] The WHI showed an increased risk for breast cancer after 3 to 5 years of combined estrogen/progestogen therapy and after 5 to 7 years of estrogen-only therapy.

Different terms are in use to describe progestogens: progesterone is the natural hormone produced in the human ovary, whereas progestins are synthetic hormones mimicking the action of the natural progesterone. Progestogen is the summarizing term for both of them.[14]

Examples for progestogen therapy with starting doses are listed in **Table 5**. Progestogens are either commercially available as combination product with estrogen, or can be individually combined with estrogens fixed or individually matched to a given estrogen dose. In order to prevent endometrial hyperplasia, progestogens should be given for at least 10 to 14 days every month.[10] Continuous progestogen exposure is not recommended per AACE guidelines, and long-cycle progestogen therapy (14 days every 3 months) may be considered in order to reduce the risk for breast cancer.[10] The progestin intrauterine device can also be used for endometrial protection, and has been shown to be equivalent or superior to systemic therapy.[15] However, it is not FDA approved for this indication.

Although progestogen-only therapy for vasomotor symptoms has been shown to be beneficial in several studies,[16,17] because of the concern of breast stimulation, ACOG and AACE do not recommend progestogen-only therapy for hot flashes.[10,18]

Progestogens without estrogens are not FDA approved for the treatment of vasomotor symptoms.

Bioidentical hormones
Patients often inquire about bioidentical hormones. This term describes custom-made formulations specifically compounded for each patient according to her physician's instructions. The term indicates that bioidentical hormones are chemically similar or structurally identical to hormones produced in the ovary. Bioidentical hormones can also contain a combination of different hormones. They can be administered via nonstandard routes such as subdermal implants or pellets, and they can contain nonhormonal ingredients (eg, dyes, preservatives) that can cause allergies in the individual using the product.

Bioidentical hormones are not FDA approved for the treatment of vasomotor symptoms. Concerns with bioidentical hormones include the following: (1) no testing for efficacy and safety, (2) uncertain purity and standardization, (3) difficult assessment of dosing, and (4) no packaging insert detailing the attributes and potential risks of the hormone product.

The lack of accurate, verifiable dosing assessment can cause problems if not enough estrogen is present to prevent the loss of bone density, or if too much estrogen and not adequate progestogen are given, with the risk for endometrial hyperplasia. ACOG, AACE, and NAMS therefore do not recommend compounded therapy unless the patient has a proven allergy to an FDA-approved formulation.[18]

How long should hormone therapy be continued?
The WHI has shown increased risk for the development of breast cancer after prolonged use. Therefore the length of treatment has to be individualized and coupled with good surveillance options for breast cancer. Up to 50% of women report recurrence of vasomotor symptoms after discontinuation of hormone therapy, regardless of age and duration of prior use.[19] Because endogenous estrogen production gradually decreases over time and with age, it seems reasonable to taper therapy. Per NAMS, the decision to continue hormone therapy should be "individualized based on the severity of symptoms and current benefit-risk ratio consideration."

Hormone therapy in postmenopausal women should not be used in order to prevent chronic conditions such as coronary artery disease or dementia,[20] unless menopause was caused by surgical intervention or premature ovarian insufficiency before the age of 50 years. Hormone therapy should not be started later than 10 years after menopause, or after age 60 years,[21] because this can put the patient at higher risk for cardiovascular events or worsening of dementia.

Nonestrogen Pharmaceutical Therapy

Selective serotonin reuptake inhibitors
SSRIs are possible alternatives to hormone therapy for the treatment of vasomotor symptoms. The exact mechanism of action for SSRIs and serotonin-norepinephrine reuptake inhibitor (SNRIs) is unknown. Both serotonin and norepinephrine can directly and indirectly influence the thermoneutral zone via a central and peripheral mechanism. The current thinking suggests that, as estrogen levels decline, norepinephrine levels increase, which causes an increase in hypothalamic serotonin receptors, and further narrowing of the thermoneutral zone. When women take SSRIs, there is an increase in serotonin levels within the brain leading to a widening of the thermoneutral zone and an improvement in vasomotor symptoms. Estrogen also stimulates alpha-2 receptors, which leads to a further increase in norepinephrine levels and, as a consequence, further narrowing of the thermoneutral zone (see **Fig. 1**). Because hot flashes

Table 5
Treatment options for vasomotor symptoms

Treatment	Dose and Administration	Evidence	FDA Approval	References
Hormonal				
Estrogen				
Ultralow dose	Transdermal estradiol 17β 0.0075 mg/d	Yes	No	54
	Transdermal estradiol 17β 0.014 mg/d	—	—	—
	Micronized estradiol 17β 0.25 mg/d orally	—	—	—
Low dose	Transdermal estradiol 17β 0.025 mg/d	Yes	Yes	55–59
	Micronized estradiol 17β 0.5 mg/d orally	—	—	—
	Conjugated equine estrogen 0.3 mg/d orally	—	—	—
Standard dose	Transdermal estradiol 17β 0.05 mg/d	Yes	Yes	55,56
	Micronized estradiol 17β 1 mg/d orally	—	—	—
	Conjugated equine estrogen 0.625 mg/d orally	—	—	—
Progestogen in combination with estrogen				
Standard dose	Medroxyprogesterone acetate 5 mg/d orally	Yes	Yes	55,56
Levonorgestrel IUD	Intrauterine levonorgestrel 20 μg/d	Yes	No	15
Estrogen + agonist/antagonist	Conjugated estrogen 0.45 mg/d + bazedoxifene 20 mg/d orally	Yes	Yes	12
Testosterone	—	No	No	32
Bioidentical hormones	Compounded	No	No	18
Progestogen only	Megestrol acetate 20 mg/d orally	Yes: prospective trial	No	16
	Depo medroxyprogesterone acetate 400 mg IM	Yes: prospective trial	No	16
Nonhormonal pharmaceutical				
SSRI	—	—	No	—

Paroxetine	7.5 mg/d orally	Yes: double blind, placebo, multicenter	Yes	24
	10–25 mg/d orally	Yes: placebo, RCT	No	7
Fluoxetine	20–30 mg/d orally	Yes: placebo, RCT	No	8
Citalopram	20–40 mg/d orally	Yes: placebo	No	25
Sertraline	25–250 mg/d orally	Yes: RCT	No	60
SNRI				
Venlafaxine	35.5–75 mg/d orally	Yes: RCT	No	61
Desvenlafaxine	100 mg/d orally	Yes: RCT	No	62
Gabapentin	900 mg/d orally	Yes: RCT	No	30
Clonidine	0.1 mg/d orally	Yes: RCT	No	63
Nonpharmaceutical				
Acupuncture	—	Yes: RCT	No	42
Exercise	—	No	No	39
Relaxation	—	No	No	38
Yoga	—	No	No	37
Black cohosh	—	Unclear	No	46,47
Phytoestrogens	—	Unclear	No	51,52
Vitamin E	800 IU/d orally	No	No	44
Omega-3 fatty acids	1.8 g/d orally	No	No	45

Abbreviations: M, intramuscular; IUD, intrauterine device; RCT, randomized controlled trial.

and depression seem to be connected, it is difficult to determine whether SSRIs help with the vasomotor symptoms, or depression, or both. All SSRIs can interfere with the metabolism of tamoxifen (Nolvadex, Soltamox) to its active metabolite endoxifen by inhibiting the cytochrome P (CYP) 450 (CYP2D6) enzyme system. This interference causes decreased efficacy of tamoxifen and can potentially increase reoccurrence of breast cancer.[22] SSRIs therefore should not be used in women taking tamoxifen. Bupropion (Wellbutrin, Zyban) as well can interfere with the CYP 450 system and therefore should also be avoided in these situations.[23]

The only FDA-approved nonhormonal formulation for hot flashes is a low dose (7.5 mg) of paroxetine (Brisdelle[24]). This dose is less than commonly used doses for the treatment of psychiatric diseases. Other higher doses the of paroxetine (Paxil, Pexeva), although not FDA approved, have been evaluated as well. Examples for other SSRIs with their starting doses are listed in **Table 5**. Direct comparison of SSRI use with estrogen is limited. Other SSRIs have shown efficacy in decreasing vasomotor symptoms as well. For example, citalopram (Celexa), an SSRI, seems to be effective for women with sleep difficulties.[25]

Selective norepinephrine reuptake inhibitors
SNRIs are only weak inhibitors of the CYP2D6 system and therefore may represent a safer alternative for women with a history of breast cancer or women who are taking tamoxifen. Examples for starting doses are listed in **Table 5**. The most common side effects of SNRIs include nausea, dizziness, and insomnia.

Clonidine
Clonidine (Catapres) is a centrally acting alpha-adrenergic agonist. Several trials have shown benefit in the treatment of hot flashes using doses of 0.1 mg orally daily, although not to the same extent as hormone therapy.[26,27] The use of clonidine is limited by its significant side effects, including dry mouth, constipation, and insomnia.

Gabapentin
Gabapentin (Neurontin) is an anticonvulsant. Its mechanism of action for vasomotor symptoms is unknown, but is thought to be related to the modulation of calcium channels. Gabapentin is a ligand of the $\alpha 2\delta 1$ and $\alpha 2\delta 2$ subunits of the voltage-gated calcium channels. The subunits increase the density of calcium channels at the plasma membrane.[28] There are no good trials available comparing gabapentin with SSRIs, and gabapentin is not as effective as hormone therapy.[29] Side effects include somnolence, disorientation, headache, and peripheral edema. Most trials evaluating gabapentin for hot flashes used a dose of 900 mg daily.[30] In one double-blinded randomized controlled trial, gabapentin in a daily dose of 2400 mg was equivalent to a standard dose (0.625 mg) of conjugated equine estrogen in alleviating hot flashes.[31]

Testosterone
Testosterone (Androderm, Testim) has not shown any benefit in the treatment of vasomotor symptoms. It has potential adverse effects, including negative effects on the lipid parameters, clitoromegaly, hirsutism, and acne.[32] Testosterone is not recommended for the treatment of hot flashes. For some postmenopausal women, it may improve sexual function scores.[33]

Tibolone
Tibolone is a synthetic steroid with tissue-specific estrogenic and progestogenic effects. It is currently not available in the United States. It has shown to have beneficial effects on vasomotor symptoms, bone mineral density, and vaginal symptoms, with

no estrogenic effect on endometrium and breast tissue. Its use has been limited by its androgenic side effects.

Nonpharmaceutical Therapy

Behavioral changes

The NAMS lists behavioral changes that can be beneficial for the treatment of mild to moderate hot flushes.[34] These changes include:

- Dressing in layers
- Consuming cold beverages and foods
- Avoiding hot and spicy foods
- Avoiding hot and alcoholic beverages
- Using a personal fan
- Smoking cessation[35]

A recent pilot study showed that losing weight helped improve the frequency of hot flashes in overweight and obese women.[36] Short-term anxiolytics such as alprazolam (Xanax, Nivaram) may help if hot flashes are caused by stressful situations.

Yoga, exercise, relaxation techniques, acupuncture

Yoga, relaxation techniques such as slow breathing, exercise, and mindfulness-based stress reduction may reduce the extent to which hot flashes interfere with a woman's daily function, although these methods have not been shown to decrease hot flashes.[37–40] Exercise can increase the severity of vasomotor symptoms in obese women, because adipose tissue acts as an insulator.[41] A recent randomized controlled trial[42] and a recent meta-analysis[43] have documented the benefit of acupuncture in decreasing daily hot flashes.

Vitamin E

Vitamin E was found to have minimal to no difference for the treatment of hot flashes compared with placebo.[44] Per NAMS, women can consider herbal remedies (eg, isoflavones or vitamin E) if desired. This suggestion is not a consensus recommendation because efficacy data are inconclusive at this point.[34]

Omega-3 fatty acids

Cohen and colleagues[45] found no effect on hot flashes after treatment with 1.8 g of omega-3 fatty acids in a randomized controlled trial over a 12-week time frame.

Black cohosh

Different studies have shown inconsistent results.[46,47] Concern exists for the development of hepatitis and myopathy with continued use of black cohosh.[48]

Phytoestrogens

Phytoestrogens are nonsteroidal components with estrogenic and sometimes antiestrogenic activity. There are 3 classes of phytoestrogens:

- Isoflavones (eg, soybeans)
- Lignans (eg, flaxseed)
- Coumestans (eg, sunflower seeds)

For all phytoestrogens, equol is the active metabolite. Setchell and colleagues[49] found that only 50% to 70% of humans are equol producers who have the intestinal microflora to transform phytoestrogens into equol. Consumption of phytoestrogens by non–equol producers may therefore have limited or no benefit. The average phytoestrogen intake in the Western world is 3 mg/d, whereas in Japan it is 50 mg/d.[50]

Overall, studies of phytoestrogens show different results[51,52] using different doses. There are no consensus recommendations, and ACOG does not recommend their use.[53]

Because it is not clear how much estrogen is generated from soy intake, women with a personal or strong family history of hormone-dependent cancers, venous thromboembolism, or cardiovascular disease should not consider soy-based treatments.[10]

VAGINAL ATROPHY/DYSPAREUNIA

Vaginal atrophy and resulting dyspareunia are late signs of the perimenopausal transition, caused by a lack of estrogen. Details about pathophysiology and guidelines for treatment are listed in **Box 2**.

LOW BONE DENSITY/OSTEOPOROSIS

Low bone density (previously called osteopenia) and osteoporosis are 5 times more common in women than in men. Information about screening, prevention, and treatment can be found in **Box 3**.

CARDIOVASCULAR DISEASE

Cardiovascular disease is the leading cause of death for women in the United States, and therefore is the most dangerous consequence of menopause. Premenopausal women producing endogenous estrogen are protected compared with men, but, after menopause, because of the lack of protective estrogen, the risk for women increases significantly. **Box 4** lists risk factors and preventative measures.

Box 2
Vaginal atrophy/dyspareunia

Hypoestrogenism causes loss of epithelial cells, loss of elasticity, loss of subcutaneous fat, and increase in vaginal pH

Common symptoms are vaginal and vulvar dryness, pruritus, dyspareunia, and vaginal infections

Treatment options:

- Water-based or silicone based vaginal lubricants (mostly used before and during intercourse)

- Any of the systemic estrogen formulations (except ultralow dose) are FDA approved for vaginal atrophy

- Local estrogen: estradiol 17β cream 2 g/d, conjugated equine estrogen cream 0.5 to 2 g/d, estradiol ring 0.05 mg/d. Ultralow dose: 17β-estradiol tablet 0.01 mg/d vaginally[64]

  Use daily for 1 to 2 weeks, then once or twice weekly for maintenance

  Theoretic concern for endometrial hyperplasia, but not proved

- Ospemifene 60 mg/d

  FDA approved for moderate-severe dyspareunia in postmenopausal women

  No stimulatory effect on endometrium[65]

  Side effects include hot flashes, vaginal discharge, and muscle spasm

Box 3
Low bone density/osteoporosis

Fastest bone loss occurs within 3 years after menopause (reduction in estrogen level increases osteoclast activity)

Recommended intake (IOM)

   Calcium 1200 mg/d and vitamin D 600 IU/d (ages 51–70 years)

   Calcium 1200 mg/d and vitamin D 800 IU/d (age 71 years and older)

DEXA bone scan recommended at age 65 years; should be performed at younger age if:

- Personal history of fragility fracture
- Smoking
- Alcohol abuse
- Body weight less than 58 kg (127 lb)
- Medical causes of bone loss: endocrine disease, gastrointestinal disease
- History of hip fracture in parents
- Rheumatoid arthritis

Lifestyle changes include:

- Regular weight-bearing exercise
- Optimization of eyesight
- Decrease fall risk in homestead

Treatment options include:

- Bisphosphonates
- SERMs (eg, Raloxifene)
- Calcitonin
- Parathyroid hormone
- Systemic estrogen

Abbreviation: IOM, Institute of Medicine.

Box 4
Cardiovascular disease

- Atherosclerosis in major vessels
- Risk factors are the same for women and men: family history, hypertension, smoking, diabetes, abnormal lipid panel, increased homocysteine level, and obesity (mainly central adiposity indicating hyperandrogenic state)
- Endothelial damage and high low-density lipoprotein–cholesterol cause foam cells, fatty streaks, and eventually atherosclerotic fibrous plaques
- Estrogen protects premenopausal women against cardiovascular disease because of vasodilatory effects (via nitric oxide) and antithrombotic effects (via prostacyclin)
- Risk for cardiovascular disease is higher in men than in premenopausal women, but after menopause risk is the same in men and women
- Estrogen given after menopause in preexisting atherosclerosis induces matrix metalloproteinase activity, which makes plaques unstable and can worsen disease
- Strongest predictor in women: high-density lipoprotein–cholesterol less than 50 mg/dL
- Decrease in risk factors is the most important preventative measure

SUMMARY/DISCUSSION

Hot flashes are primarily caused by a decrease in estrogen levels and change in neurotransmitters occurring during the menopausal transition, leading to narrowing of the thermoneutral zone. Known risk factors include ethnicity, obesity, and cigarette smoking. The most effective treatment of hot flashes is hormone therapy using estrogen with or without a progestogen depending on the presence of a uterus, followed by nonhormonal pharmacologic therapies (SSRIs, SNRIs, clonidine, gabapentin) and nonpharmacologic therapy options (behavioral changes, acupuncture). The major risks associated with hormone therapy include development of breast cancer, venous thromboembolism, and cerebrovascular disease. Hormone therapy is not indicated for the prevention of chronic conditions. SSRIs should not be used in women with a history of breast cancer, or women who are taking tamoxifen. The best treatment option for vasomotor symptoms often is individualized therapy for each patient.

REFERENCES

1. Thurston RC, Joffe H. Vasomotor symptoms and menopause: findings from the Study of Women's Health across the Nation. Obstet Gynecol Clin North Am 2011;38:489–501.
2. Sturdee DW. The menopausal hot flush – anything new? Maturitas 2008;60:42–9.
3. Crandall CJ, Crawford SL, Gold EB. Vasomotor symptom prevalence is associated with polymorphisms in sex steroid-metabolizing enzymes and receptors. Am J Med 2006;119:S52–60.
4. Pachman DR, Jones JM, Loprinzi CL. Management of menopause-associated vasomotor symptoms: current treatment options, challenges and future directions. Int J Womens Health 2010;2:123–35.
5. Dalal S, Zhukovsky DS. Pathophysiology and management of hot flashes. J Support Oncol 2006;4:315–20.
6. Freedman RR. Pathophysiology and treatment of menopausal hot flashes. Semin Reprod Med 2005;23:117–25.
7. Shanafelt TD, Barton DL, Adjei AA, et al. Pathophysiology and treatment of hot flashes. Mayo Clin Proc 2002;77:1207–18.
8. Sowers MR, Wilson AL, Karvonen-Gutierrez CA, et al. Sex steroid hormone pathway genes and health-related measures in women of 4 races/ethnicities: the Study of Women's Health Across the Nation (SWAN). Am J Med 2006;119: S103–10.
9. Laliberte F, Dea K, Duh MS, et al. Does the route of administration for estrogen hormone therapy impact the risk of venous thromboembolism? Estradiol transdermal system versus oral estrogen-only hormone therapy. Menopause 2011; 18:1052–9.
10. American Association of Clinical Endocrinologists (AACE) medical guidelines for clinical practice for the diagnosis and treatment of menopause 2011. National Guideline Clearinghouse (NGC) 008903.
11. MacLennan AH, Henry D, Hills S, et al. Oral oestrogen replacement therapy versus placebo for hot flushes. Cochrane Database of Systematic Reviews 2001;(1):CD002978.
12. Lobo RA, Pinkerton JV, Gass ML, et al. Evaluation of bazedoxifene/conjugated estrogens for the treatment of menopausal symptoms and effects on metabolic parameters and overall safety profile. Fertil Steril 2009;92:1025–38.
13. Hofseth LJ, Raafat AM, Osuch JR, et al. Hormone replacement therapy with estrogen or estrogen plus medroxyprogesterone acetate is associated with

increased epithelial proliferation in the normal postmenopausal breast. J Clin Endocrinol Metab 1999;84:4559–65.

14. Romero R, Stanczyk FZ. Progesterone is not the same as 17α-hydroxyprogesterone caproate: implications for obstetrical practice. Am J Obstet Gynecol 2013; 208:421–6.

15. Somboonporn W, Panna S, Temtanakitpaisan T, et al. Effects of the levonorgestrel-releasing intrauterine system plus estrogen therapy in perimenopausal and postmenopausal women: systematic review and meta-analysis. Menopause 2011;18: 1060–6.

16. Bertelli G, Venturini M, Del Mastro L, et al. Intramuscular depot medroxyprogesterone versus oral megestrol for the control of postmenopausal hot flashes in breast cancer patients: a randomized study. Ann Oncol 2002;13:883–8.

17. Loprinzi CL, Michalak JC, Quella SK, et al. Megestrol acetate for the prevention of hot flashes. N Engl J Med 1994;331:347–52.

18. Committee on Gynecologic Practice and the American Society for Reproductive Medicine Practice Committee American College of Obstetricians and Gynecologists. Committee opinion no. 532: compounded bioidentical menopausal hormone therapy. Obstet Gynecol 2012;120:411–5.

19. Brunner RL, Aragaki A, Barnabei V, et al. Menopausal symptom experience before and after stopping estrogen therapy in the Women's Health Initiative randomized, placebo-controlled trial. Menopause 2010;17:946–54.

20. Moyer VA, U.S. Preventive Services Task Force. Menopausal hormone therapy for the primary prevention of chronic conditions: U.S. Preventive Services Task Force Recommendations statement. Ann Intern Med 2013;158:47–54.

21. Salpeter SR, Walsh JM, Greyber E, et al. Mortality associated with hormone replacement therapy in younger and older women. J Gen Intern Med 2004;19:791–804.

22. Kelly CM, Juurlink DN, Gomes T, et al. Selective serotonin reuptake inhibitors and breast cancer mortality in women receiving tamoxifen: a population based cohort study. BMJ 2010;340:c693.

23. Desmarais JE, Looper KJ. Managing menopausal symptoms and depression in tamoxifen users: implications of drug and medicinal interactions. Maturitas 2010;67:296–308.

24. Simon JA, Portman DJ, Kaunitz AM, et al. Low-dose paroxetine 7.5 mg for menopausal vasomotor symptoms: two randomized controlled trials. Menopause 2013; 20:1027–35.

25. Kalay AE, Demir B, Haberal A, et al. Efficacy of citalopram on climacteric symptoms. Menopause 2007;13:223–9.

26. Nelson HD, Vesco KK, Haney E, et al. Nonhormonal therapies for menopausal hot flashes: systematic review and meta-analysis. JAMA 2006;295:2057–71.

27. Pandya KJ, Raubertas RF, Flynn PJ, et al. Oral clonidine in postmenopausal patients with breast cancer experiencing tamoxifen-induced hot flashes: a University of Rochester Cancer Centre Community Clinical Oncology Program Study. Ann Intern Med 2000;132:788–93.

28. Davies A, Hendrich J, Van Minh AT. Functional biology of the alpha(2)delta subunits of voltage-gated calcium channels. Trends Pharmacol Sci 2007;28:220–8.

29. Aguirre W, Chedraui P, Mendoza J, et al. Gabapentin vs. low-dose transdermal estradiol for treating post-menopausal women with moderate to very severe hot flushes. Gynecol Endocrinol 2010;26:333–7.

30. Guttoso T Jr, Kurlan R, McDermott MP, et al. Gabapentin's effect on hot flashes in postmenopausal women; a randomized controlled trial. Obstet Gynecol 2003; 101:337–45.

31. Reddy SY, Warner H, Guttoso T Jr, et al. Gabapentin, estrogen, and placebo for treating hot flushes: a randomized controlled trial. Obstet Gynecol 2006;108: 41–8.

32. Matthews KA, Owens JF, Salomon K, et al. Influence of hormone therapy on the cardiovascular responses to stress of postmenopausal women. Biol Psychol 2005;69:39–56.

33. Somboonporn W, Davis S, Seif MW, et al. Testosterone for peri- and postmeno-pausal women. Cochrane Database Syst Rev 2005;(4):CD004509.

34. North American Menopause Society. The 2012 hormone therapy position state-ment of the North American Menopause Society. Menopause 2012;19:257–71.

35. National Guideline Clearinghouse. Vasomotor symptoms. In: menopause and osteoporosis update 2009. J Obstet Gynaecol Can 2009;31:S9–10.

36. Thurston RC, Ewing LJ, Low CA, et al. Behavioral weight loss for the management of menopausal hot flashes: a pilot study. Menopause 2014. [Epub ahead of print].

37. Reed SD, Guthrie KA, Newton KM, et al. Menopausal quality of life: RCT of yoga, exercise, and omega-3 supplements. Am J Obstet Gynecol 2014;210:244.e1–11.

38. Nedstrand E, Wijma K, Wyon Y, et al. Applied relaxation and oral estradiol treat-ment of vasomotor symptoms in postmenopausal women. Maturitas 2005;51: 154–62.

39. Sternfeld B, Guthrie KA, Ensrud KE, et al. Efficacy of exercise for menopausal symptoms: a randomized controlled trial. Menopause 2014;21:330–8.

40. Carmody JF, Crawford S, Salmoirago-Blotcher E, et al. Mindfulness training for coping with hot flashes: results of a randomized trial. Menopause 2011;18: 611–20.

41. Lindh-Astrand L, Nedstrand E, Wyon Y, et al. Vasomotor symptoms and quality of life in previously sedentary postmenopausal women randomized to physical ac-tivity or estrogen therapy. Maturitas 2004;48:97–105.

42. Richard-Davis G. Are acupuncture and Chinese herbal medicine effective op-tions for hot flashes? Menopause 2014;21:3–5.

43. Chiu HY, Pan CH, Shyu YK, et al. Effects of acupuncture on menopause-related symptoms and quality of life in women on natural menopause: a meta-analysis of randomized controlled trials. Menopause 2014. [Epub ahead of print].

44. Loprinzi CL, Barton DL, Sloan JA, et al. Mayo Clinic and North Central Cancer treatment group hot flash studies: a 20-year experience. Menopause 2008;15: 655–60.

45. Cohen LS, Joffe H, Guthrie KA, et al. Efficacy of omega-3 for vasomotor symp-toms treatment: a randomized controlled trial. Menopause 2014;21:347–54.

46. Newton KM, Reed SD, LaCroix AZ, et al. Treatment of vasomotor symptoms of menopause with black cohosh, multibotanicals, soy, hormone therapy, or placebo. Ann Intern Med 2006;145:869–79.

47. Nedrow A, Miller J, Walker M, et al. Complementary and alternative therapies for the management of menopause-related symptoms. Arch Intern Med 2006;166: 1453–65.

48. Teschke R, Schwarzenboeck A, Schmidt-Taenzer W, et al. Herb induced liver injury presumably caused by black cohosh: a survey of initially purported cases and herbal quality specifications. Ann Hepatol 2011;10:249–59.

49. Setchell KD, Brown NM, Lydeking-Olsen E. The clinical importance of the metab-olite equol–a clue to the effectiveness of soy and its isoflavones. J Nutr 2002;132: 3557–84.

50. Messina M. Isoflavone intakes by Japanese were overestimated. Am J Clin Nutr 1995;62:64.

51. Han KK, Soares JM, Haidar MA, et al. Benefits of soy isoflavone therapeutic regimen on menopausal symptoms. Obstet Gynecol 2002;99:389–94.
52. St. Germain A, Peterson CT, Robinson JG, et al. Isoflavone-rich or isoflavone-poor soy protein does not reduce menopausal symptoms during 24 weeks of treatment. Menopause 2001;8:17–26.
53. Clinical Management Guidelines for Obstetrician-Gynecologists. Management of menopausal symptoms. Obstet Gynecol 2014;123:202–16.
54. Mørch LS, Løkkegaard E, Andreasen AH, et al. Hormone therapy and ovarian cancer. JAMA 2009;302:298–305.
55. Bachmann GA, Schaefers M, Uddin A, et al. Lowest effective transdermal 17beta-estradiol dose for relief of hot flashes in postmenopausal women: a randomized controlled trial. Obstet Gynecol 2007;110:771–9.
56. MacLennan AH, Broadbent JL, Lester S, et al. Oral oestrogen and combined oestrogen/progestogen therapy versus placebo for hot flushes. Cochrane Database of Systematic Reviews 2004;(4):CD002978.
57. Greendale GA, Reboussin BA, Hogan P, et al. Symptom relief and side effects of postmenopausal hormones: results from the Postmenopausal Estrogen/Progestin Interventions Trial. Obstet Gynecol 1998;92:982–8.
58. Soares CN, Joffe H, Viguera AC, et al. Paroxetine versus placebo for women in midline after hormone therapy discontinuation. Am J Med 2008;121:159–62.e1.
59. Oktem M, Eroglu D, Karahan HB, et al. Black cohosh and fluoxetine in the treatment of postmenopausal symptoms: a prospective, randomized trial. Adv Ther 2007;24:448–61.
60. Gordon PR, Kerwin JP, Boesen KG, et al. Sertraline to treat hot flashes: a randomized controlled, double-blind, crossover trial in a general population. Menopause 2006;13:568–75.
61. Evans MI, Pritts E, Vittinghoff E, et al. Management of postmenopausal hot flushes with venlafaxine hydrochloride: a randomized controlled trial. Obstet Gynecol 2005;105:161–6.
62. Archer DF, Seidman L, Constantine GD, et al. A double blind, randomly assigned, placebo-controlled study of desvenlafaxine efficacy and safety for the treatment of vasomotor symptoms associated with menopause. Am J Obstet Gynecol 2009; 200:172.e1–10.
63. Goldberg RM, Loprinzi CL, O'Fallon JR, et al. Transdermal clonidine for ameliorating tamoxifen-induced hot flashes. J Clin Oncol 1994;12:155–8.
64. Simon J, Nachtigall L, Gut R, et al. Effective treatment of vaginal atrophy with an ultra-low-dose estradiol vaginal tablet. Obstet Gynecol 2008;112:1053–60.
65. Bachmann GA, Komi JO. Ospemifene effectively treats vulvovaginal atrophy in postmenopausal women: results from a pivotal phase 3 study. Ospemifene study group. Menopause 2010;17:480–6.

Index

Note: Page numbers of article titles are in **boldface** type.

A

Abdominal myomectomy
  in leiomyoma management, 77
Abnormal uterine bleeding (AUB)
  described, 103–105
  normal menstrual bleeding *vs.,* 104–105
  in reproductive-aged women, **103–115**
    discussion of, 113
    evaluation of, 105–108
      history and physical examination in, 105–106
      laboratory testing in, 106–107
      uterine-related, 107–108
    introduction, 103–104
    management of, 108–113
      antifibrinolytics in, 112
      hormonal therapies in, 109–111
      medical, 108–112
      NSAIDs in, 111–112
      surgical therapies in, 112–113
Acne
  hyperandrogenism and, 58–59
Acupuncture
  in hot flashes management, 173
Age at menarche
  leiomyoma related to, 68
Age-related infertility, **15–25**
  discussion, 16–21
  introduction, 15–16
  maternal and fetal risks associated with, 21
  ovarian reserve management and treatment, 18–21
  ovarian reserve testing, 17–18
  physiology of reproductive aging, 16–17
Aging
  reproductive
    physiology of, 16–17
Alloimmune factors
  RPL related to, 123
Aneuploidy
  miscarriage and, 125
Anovulation
  clomiphene citrate–resistant
    exogenous gonadotropins for, 33

Obstet Gynecol Clin N Am 42 (2015) 181–192
http://dx.doi.org/10.1016/S0889-8545(15)00011-X
0889-8545/15/$ – see front matter © 2015 Elsevier Inc. All rights reserved.

obgyn.theclinics.com

Printed and bound by CPI Group (UK) Ltd, Croydon, CR0 4YY

03/10/2024

01040495-0019